Understanding the I

The Functional Gastroi

OTHER BOOKS BY DR. W. GRANT THOMPSON

Thompson WG. *The Irritable Gut: Functional Disorders of the Alimentary Canal.* Baltimore: University Park Press; 1979.

Thompson WG. *Gut Reactions: Understanding Symptoms of the Digestive Tract.* New York: Plenum Publishing; 1989.

Thompson WG. *The Angry Gut: Coping with Colitis and Crohn's Disease.* New York: Plenum Publishing; 1993.

Drossman DA, Richter JE, Talley NJ, Thompson WG, Corazziari E, Whitehead WE. *Functional Gastrointestinal Disorders.* Boston: Little, Brown, and Company; 1994. Reprinted McLean, VA: Degnon Associates, Inc.; 1997.

Thompson WG. *The Ulcer Story: The Authoritative Guide to Ulcers, Dyspepsia, and Heartburn.* New York: Plenum Publishing; 1996.

Heaton KW, Thompson WG. *Fast Facts: Irritable Bowel Syndrome.* Oxford: Health Press; 1999.

Drossman DA, Corazziari E, Talley NJ, Thompson WG, Whitehead WE. *Rome II: The Functional Gastrointestinal Disorders.* McLean, VA: Degnon Associates, Inc.; 2000.

Thompson WG, Heaton KW. *Fast Facts: Irritable Bowel Syndrome*, 2nd ed. Oxford: Health Press; 2003.

Thompson WG. *The Placebo Effect: Combining Science and Compassionate Care.* Amherst, NY: Prometheus Books; 2005.

Drossman DA, Corazziari E, Delvaux M, Talley NJ, Spiller RC, Thompson WG, Whitehead WE. *Rome III: The Functional Gastrointestinal Disorders.* McLean, VA: Degnon Associates, Inc.; 2006.

Understanding the Irritable Gut
The Functional Gastrointestinal Disorders

W. GRANT THOMPSON, MD

Edited by Douglas A. Drossman, MD

A Rome Foundation Educational Product
Published by Degnon Associates, McLean, Virginia

Copyright © 2008 by the Rome Foundation

All rights reserved. No part of this book may be reproduced in any form or by electronic or mechanical means, including information storage and retrieval systems, without permission in writing from the publisher, except by a reviewer who may quote brief passages in a review.

Copy editor, Diane Feldman
Illustrator, Jerry Schoendorf
Designer, Julie Allred, BW&A Books, Inc.
Printer, Edwards Brothers, Inc.

This book is printed on acid-free paper. According to the Environmental Defense Fund Paper Calculator, using this 100% recycled paper saved 144 mature trees. ✪

ISBN: 978-0-9656837-8-4
Library of Congress Control Number: 2008929286

Printed in the United States of America
First Edition
First Printing

Contents

Editor's Note *vii*

Foreword A Doctor's View *ix*

Foreword A Patient's View *xiii*

Preface The Basis of This Book: The Work of the Rome Foundation to Improve the Lives of Patients with Functional GI Disorders *xv*

Acknowledgments *xix*

PART 1 About the Functional Gastrointestinal Disorders

Introduction *1*

1 What Are the Functional Gastrointestinal Disorders? *3*

2 How Common Are the Functional Gastrointestinal Disorders? *12*

3 The Gut: How It Works *20*

4 What Causes the Functional Gastrointestinal Disorders? *32*

PART 2 The Functional Gastrointestinal Disorders: Nature and Diagnosis

Introduction *41*

5 How Are the Functional Gastrointestinal Disorders Diagnosed? *43*

6 Irritable Bowel Syndrome *49*

7 Functional Constipation *60*

8 Functional Diarrhea *68*

9 Functional Dyspepsia (Nonulcer Dyspepsia) *74*

10 Heartburn, Chest Pain, Dysphagia: The Functional Esophageal Disorders *82*

11 Incontinence, Anal Pain, Defecation Disorders: The Functional Anorectal Disorders *88*

vi Contents

12 Belching, Bloating, Pain, and the Other Functional Gastrointestinal Disorders *94*

PART 3 **Managing the Functional Gastrointestinal Disorders**

Introduction *107*

13 General Treatment Measures *108*

14 The Therapeutic Relationship: Doctors, Patients, and the Placebo Effect *116*

15 Proving Treatments Work: Randomized Clinical Trials *127*

16 Management of the Functional Gastrointestinal Disorders *142*

17 Treatments *163*

Epilogue The Challenges *177*

Appendix A The *Rome III* Diagnostic Criteria for the Functional Gastrointestinal Disorders *183*

Appendix B Some Tests Commonly Used in the Investigation of the Functional Gastrointestinal Disorders *200*

Glossary *207*

Resources *225*

Index *227*

Editor's Note

The mission of the Rome Foundation is "To improve the lives of patients with functional GI disorders." Thus, it is with pride and gratitude that the foundation supports this book, *Understanding the Irritable Gut,* written by Dr. Grant Thompson. Dr. Thompson, a member of the Rome Foundation board and a pioneer in the area of functional GI disorders, is well recognized for his knowledge of the field and for his superb writing skills. He is an ideal person to "translate" in a nontechnical fashion the evolving information that is offered in our book for professionals: *Rome III: The Functional Gastrointestinal Disorders.*

The Rome organization, now nearly twenty years old, is committed to helping clinicians, scientists, industry, federal agencies, and the general public understand the functional gastrointestinal disorders. In addition to creating and revising the *Rome* diagnostic criteria, we seek to consolidate and disseminate the wealth of knowledge that exists in our field, and to legitimize these disorders to patients and professionals alike. For doctors, this occurs through our international publications, our Web site (www.theromecriteria.org), our large and growing series of educational presentations at meetings around the world, and in our financial support for research studies. We have developed widely accepted recommendations for the design of treatment trials to enable the development of new pharmaceutical agents, and we collaborate with national and international organizations to maintain the high educational and training standards needed for the growth of this discipline. For other health care personnel and the public, this book is our first educational resource. It results from our decision to disseminate the growing knowledge of the functional GI disorders to the general public and to non-gastroenterologist health care professionals.

We are grateful to our sponsors who have generously supported our efforts: AstraZeneca International, Axcan Pharma, Inc., Forest Research Institute, GlaxoSmithKline, Ortho-McNeil Pharmaceutical, Ironwood Pharmaceuticals, Inc., Procter & Gamble Pharmaceuticals, Prometheus Laboratories, Inc., Sanofi-Aventis Group, Sucampo Pharmaceuticals, Inc., and Takeda Pharmaceuticals North America.

We hope readers will find this book both interesting and informative.

Douglas A. Drossman, MD
President, Rome Foundation

Dr. Drossman is a consultant for Ironwood Pharmaceuticals, Inc., Lexicon Pharmaceuticals, Ortho-McNeil Pharmaceutical, Prometheus Laboratories, Inc., Sucampo Pharmaceuticals, Inc., and Takeda Pharmaceuticals North America.

FOREWORD
A Doctor's View

I am honored by Dr. Thompson's request to provide a perspective on how the reader can help make the patient-physician relationship meaningful. In recent years, this has become an important issue. With the emphasis over the last several decades on the use of modern technology for diagnosis, and the financial incentive for "rapid throughput" (that is, to see patients quickly to maximize reimbursement), we are at risk of losing the "patient" from patient care.

As a clinician with a lifelong career of caring for patients with functional GI disorders, I have learned that establishing a collaborative relationship is the key to attaining treatment benefit. This requires that the physician and patient mutually define their objectives and responsibilities. The goal is to partner in gaining insight into the patient's illness and disease, and use that information to establish and maintain the patient's well-being. Each has a responsibility to communicate their ideas effectively and to work toward understanding the other's ideas. Although these ideals may seem implicit, in fact they are not. Without this understanding both parties can end up dissatisfied with the provision of care and the very relationship that supports it. I've heard many patients say, "My doctor . . . doesn't listen to me," or ". . . doesn't believe what I say," or ". . . just doesn't seem to have the time." Conversely, I have heard doctors say, "My patient . . . doesn't understand what I'm trying to do," or ". . . talks about all sorts of things and doesn't focus on the treatment," or even ". . . doesn't seem interested in getting better." How can two individuals meeting presumably for the same reason see things so differently?

To understand this failure in communication, we must recognize that within medicine and gastroenterology, diagnosis is constructed primarily from a disease-based* classification system. So physicians are familiar with

---

* I make the distinction here between *disease*—evidence for structural abnormalities or disease pathology—and *illness*—the patient's perception of ill health. Although it can be assumed that disease and illness coexist, that is not always the case. With functional GI disorders in particular, there are no structural abnormalities seen on endoscopy or x-ray, and laboratory studies are normal. The symptoms are based on dysregulation of intestinal movements (motility), increased sensitivity of the nerves in the bowel (visceral hypersensitivity), and alterations in the regulation of activity between the brain and the gut.

identifying and treating ulcers, inflammatory bowel disease, diverticulitis, or cancer because the diagnosis is evident from the studies, the treatments are straightforward, and progress can be gauged by resolution of the abnormalities found on the studies (even independent of what the patients feel). Thus, the patient contributes little more to the relationship than the reporting of their symptoms. Also, doctors may not be as familiar with the newer scientific knowledge about brain-gut physiology, visceral sensitivity, altered mucosal immunity, or the role of bacteria in gut health, all of which explain the symptoms, but which are not "seen" by traditional diagnostic methods. Finally, physicians may not always be sufficiently trained in communication skills: to listen actively to their patients and attend to their concerns and needs, as well as to educate and care. Unfortunately, this "art" of medicine is becoming supplanted by the focus on technology, which places diagnosing and treating patients with functional GI disorders at a disadvantage.

Consider then what may occur in a clinical visit. Patients are encouraged to report their symptoms, but not their personal perspective on the illness, and so some questions and concerns may not be fully addressed. A doctor working from the disease-based model may do some tests but, failing to find positive results and without sufficient knowledge of these disorders, may focus on more studies to find the "cause" or may paradoxically dismiss the symptoms as trivial, or "in the head," and possibly give up responsibility for a patient's care.

Good clinicians use their knowledge of disease as a resource, but focus their attention primarily on the patient and his illness, i.e., the symptoms and associated thoughts and feelings. Using this knowledge, the doctor places it into a medical framework, makes a proper diagnosis and, when needed, performs studies. The diagnosis of functional GI disorders is vastly aided through the use of the *Rome* criteria, which are based on the specific symptoms that patients experience and report. In this way a positive diagnosis can be made, which is reassuring to patient and physician alike. Ultimately, the agenda can then move toward proper management.

Thus it is important for patients to select doctors who are interested and knowledgeable about functional GI disorders and their patients; with them diagnosis and care is optimal. It is possible to identify well-qualified physicians through organizations like the International Foundation for Functional GI Disorders (www.iffgd.org). (See the companion foreword by Nancy Norton, IFFGD president.) Individuals might also contact a medical practice and specifically ask if there are physicians who are interested in treating functional GI disorders.

Patients can also educate their physicians. If doctors operate from the belief that patients want to be "tested and treated" to find a "cure," they may feel disappointed when the studies are negative, and even display frustration or annoyance. However, with chronic illness, cure is rare. Patients need to recognize how to establish more realistic goals, to work with a doctor who is committed to ongoing care, to receive hope, and to not feel abandoned. This can begin by bringing to the first visit a clear set of manageable goals and expectations. The physician should make a diagnosis as best as possible, and then patient and doctor should work together toward improving symptoms with management (including self-management) strategies. It is a shared effort where the process of care helps the patient find ways to regain a sense of control over the illness; it also offloads from the physician the need to take on too much responsibility in the care. Patients also need to convey information in as clear a way as possible and to take the initiative to ask questions. Sometimes creating a list in advance may help. It is important to be open to the doctor's views, to respect the visit time and to phone in with questions only if they are of an urgent nature. Finally, it is important to communicate one's views of the relationship, if it is working or not working and why.

Most all doctors want to help. People who have functional GI disorders and their doctors can work together as partners to strive for optimal care.

Douglas A. Drossman, MD
Co-Director, UNC Center for Functional GI
and Motility Disorders
University of North Carolina at Chapel Hill
June 2008

FOREWORD
A Patient's View

The illness experience traditionally has been studied from the point of view of the physician observer, not the patient. Therefore, being asked to provide a patient perspective of the work of the Rome Foundation for this book is a unique honor.

Functional gastrointestinal disorders include a host of chronic conditions with symptoms that are difficult to discuss, not only with a family member or friend, but even with a medical expert. Having a chronic gastrointestinal disorder places daily challenges on the individual. The person often cannot predict symptom onset or identify all the possible trigger factors. It can mean living with daily uncertainty, which adds to the burden of the illness itself. Individuals who suffer with these disorders often go to great lengths to hide their condition from others, gradually resulting in social withdrawal. The demands placed on people with these disorders are always present, touching on virtually every aspect of their lives.

An element of stigmatization is still attached to bowel disorders. Having a stigmatized condition or diagnosis raises the possibility that the person with the disorder will be devalued by others. In response, individuals may develop strategies to cope, incorporating avoidance, withdrawal, vigilance, and concealment into their daily lives. The degree to which these strategies are applied may vary from person to person; each has an associated cost that further contributes to the social isolation or frustration felt by patients.

Although we have seen an increase in awareness of and education about the functional GI disorders over the past decade, in general the public remains ill-informed about digestive health and disease. Awareness can break down the myths and misconceptions about these disorders. However, increased awareness doesn't necessarily make it any easier to speak about symptoms, nor reduce the toll that such a disorder takes on the patient physically, socially, or professionally.

It is currently thought that as many as 70% of individuals with symptoms that are indicative of irritable bowel syndrome (IBS) do not seek medical attention. Many people are self-treating with over-the-counter medication, with not a lot of success. They are attempting to manage their condition without seeking medical attention. Many of them are misinformed about their symptoms. Their understanding of their own health problems is influenced by everyday experiences as well as by cultural, social, and media interactions, rather than by sound medical advice.

A person with IBS who does seek health care will find that his condition lacks the specificity of an acute illness with a known etiology and is often viewed as having an ambiguous identity. The patient may then discontinue seeing a physician despite the persistence of his symptoms and struggle to manage his own symptoms over the long-term course of the disorder.

For the patient with a functional GI disorder, the patient-physician relationship is fundamental to successful management of the condition. In general patients are not health experts and often do not know how or what to ask their physicians. They tend to give inconsistent accounts of their symptom experience and their bodily functions. The physician must listen carefully, ask questions, and assure the patient that he is being taken seriously. The first step toward treatment is a clear and positive explanation about the disorder. An unsatisfactory explanation may be experienced as a denial of the legitimacy of his reported symptoms, an implication that negative test results imply an absence of real disease, and a lack of understanding of or belief in his suffering. The lack of a clear medical explanation may be transformed into a personal failing on the patient's part.

There are no universally applied diagnostic criteria of the functional GI disorders. Although the means to make a positive diagnosis are available through the *Rome* criteria, we know that only a portion of physicians are aware of them and are using them. The application of experiential clinical understanding then varies depending upon the physician's knowledge and biases. Thus, patients seeking clear explanations may encounter uncertain or even conflicting views from one clinician to another.

There are many different facets to the patient perspective and a myriad of things that confound each person's experience. Knowing how to manage a chronic illness is not an innate quality—it must be taught. Patients need information relevant to their daily lives, not only about what is wrong, but also about how the condition will influence their day-to-day functioning.

A strong doctor-patient relationship requires routinely assessing problems and accomplishments, regular follow-up, and a clinician and staff who are accessible, empathetic, and knowledgeable.

Nancy Norton
President
International Foundation for Functional
  Gastrointestinal Disorders
August 2007

PREFACE

The Basis of This Book: The Work of the Rome Foundation to Improve the Lives of Patients with Functional GI Disorders

At the first-ever international symposium on the irritable bowel syndrome (IBS) at the 1984 *International Congress of Gastroenterology* in Lisbon, Portugal, I chaired a panel of experts from France, Portugal, Sweden, and Italy. Such was the physician interest in this very common but neglected disorder that the audience overfilled a small lecture hall that normally accommodated 500 people. Before then, little scientific attention had been paid to functional gastrointestinal disorders (FGIDs). The symptoms of IBS and related conditions were poorly defined and there were neither agreed-upon diagnostic techniques nor evidence-based treatments.

One panel member, Professor Aldo Torsoli, was the president of the subsequent *International Congress* to be held in Rome in 1988. Noting the curiosity of our audience and the lack of medical consensus about IBS, he commissioned me to chair a working team to prepare *Guidelines for the Management of IBS* for presentation in Rome. This working team included Gerhard Dotevall (Sweden), Douglas Drossman (US), Kenneth Heaton (UK), Wolfgang Kruis (Germany), and me from Canada. We corresponded for two years and met in Rome in 1987 to draft the guidelines.

Our work was submitted to nineteen peers from around the world whose constructive criticism was incorporated in the document. The guidelines included suggestions—not yet criteria—for diagnosis. The notion of diagnostic criteria proved to be the most important challenge, because doctors defined IBS in diverse ways. Hitherto, it was a diagnosis that was finally made after exclusion of every other possible cause.

Following the Rome congress, Professor Torsoli asked Doug Drossman to develop a classification and clinical approach for all of the functional gastrointestinal disorders, including such disparate syndromes as globus, dyspepsia, IBS, constipation, and proctalgia fugax. He assigned working teams to deal with functional disorders that were thought to originate in the esophagus, gastroduodenum, biliary tree, intestines, and anorectum. The working teams' reports appeared in the journal *Gastroenterology International* over several years and eventually in 1994 in a book—the first edition of *The Functional Gastrointestinal Disorders*. These reports included symptom criteria for the diagnosis of the disorders—the *Rome I* criteria.

At last, there was serious discussion of the FGIDs. Physicians could now make a confident diagnosis for most patients on the basis of a clinical interview and examination, rather than arriving at one after exhaustive, expensive, and sometimes dangerous testing. Properly designed randomized clinical trials became possible and researchers could report data from studies that recruited patients according to clearly defined criteria. Doctors could now apply the results of such studies to similar patients in their practices. Evidence-based medicine finally embraced the FGIDs.

Over the past twenty years, the Rome process has become more sophisticated. Figure F-1 demonstrates the rapid increase in IBS research publications since then. Successive Rome publications include the conclusions of expert working teams that address the burgeoning physiological, pharmacological, and psychosocial information about the FGIDs. Moreover, these reports review the medical evidence underpinning the recognition and proper management of these disorders. The Rome Foundation was established after the *Rome II* book was published in 2000, complete with a board, an Executive Director, George Degnon, and an Administrative Coordinator, Carlar Blackman. The process is supported by generous "arms-length" grants from the phar-

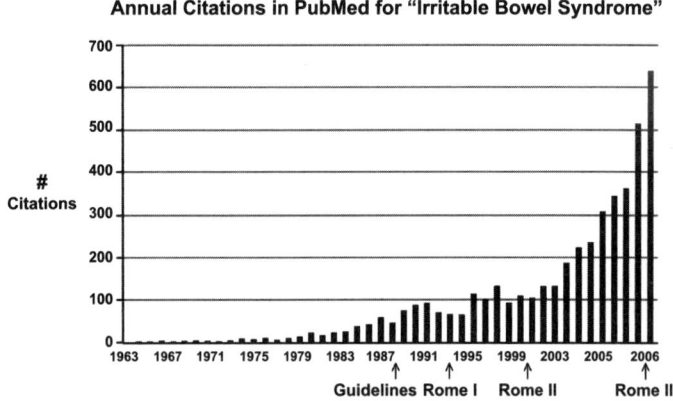

Figure F-1. Annual results of PubMed literature searches for irritable bowel syndrome and irritable colon syndrome between the 1962 Chaudhary and Truelove report and 2006. Note the rapid rise in publications as the *Rome* documents appeared. In the 1960s, half the articles had "irritable colon syndrome" in their titles; the term is rarely used now. (Adapted from *Rome III: The Functional Gastrointestinal Disorders*, p. 859.)

maceutical industry. An Industry Advisory Council, first chaired by William Whitehead and now by Lin Chang, permits annual interaction of the Rome Foundation's board with industry and regulatory representatives. Board members report to the council on the progress of the foundation's many projects without compromising the scientific deliberations of the working teams. The foundation's activities, in addition to the scientific publications and criteria development, include a compact-disc teaching project, an educational Web site (www.theromefoundation.org), the funding of research projects, and the commissioning of special working teams and symposia that address scientific issues such as clinical trial outcomes, symptom severity, and brain imaging.

The Rome process owes much to the energy and commitment of Doug Drossman and other board members who manage the foundation's ongoing activities. *Rome III: The Functional Gastrointestinal Disorders* was published in 2006. It is a valuable compendium for professionals and researchers working with patients who have these disorders. *(To order a copy, see page xviii.)*

Understanding the Irritable Gut is designed to explain the elements of *Rome III* to health professionals and the public. In their forewords to this book, Dr. Drossman, president of the Rome Foundation, and Ms. Nancy Norton, president of the International Foundation for the Functional Gastrointestinal Disorders provide doctors' and patients' perspectives. The book itself is divided into three parts, each beginning with a short introduction. Part 1 provides basic information necessary to understand the FGIDs. Part 2 describes the FGIDs themselves and their diagnosis, and part 3 their treatment. For more information readers may refer to the *Rome III* book itself, or to source material listed after each chapter in this book, or to the organizations and books listed in the Resources section.

W. Grant Thompson, MD
Ottawa, Canada
June 2008

Sources

Drossman DA, Funch-Jensen P, Janssens J, Talley NJ, Thompson WG, Whitehead WE. Identification of subgroups of functional bowel disorders. *Gastroent Int.* 1990;3:159-172.

Drossman DA, Richter JE, Talley NJ, Corazziari E, Thompson WG, Whitehead WE. *Functional Gastrointestinal Disorders.* Boston: Little, Brown, and Company; 1994.

Drossman DA, Corazziari E, Delvaux M, Spiller RC, Talley NJ, Thompson WG, Whitehead WE. *Rome III: The Functional Gastrointestinal Disorders.* McLean, VA: Degnon Associates, Inc; 2006.

Miller J, Petrie J. Development of practice guidelines. *Lancet.* 2000;355:82-83.

Thompson WG, Dotevall G, Drossman DA, Heaton KW, Kruis W. Irritable bowel syndrome: guidelines for the diagnosis. *Gastroent Int.* 1989;2:92-95.

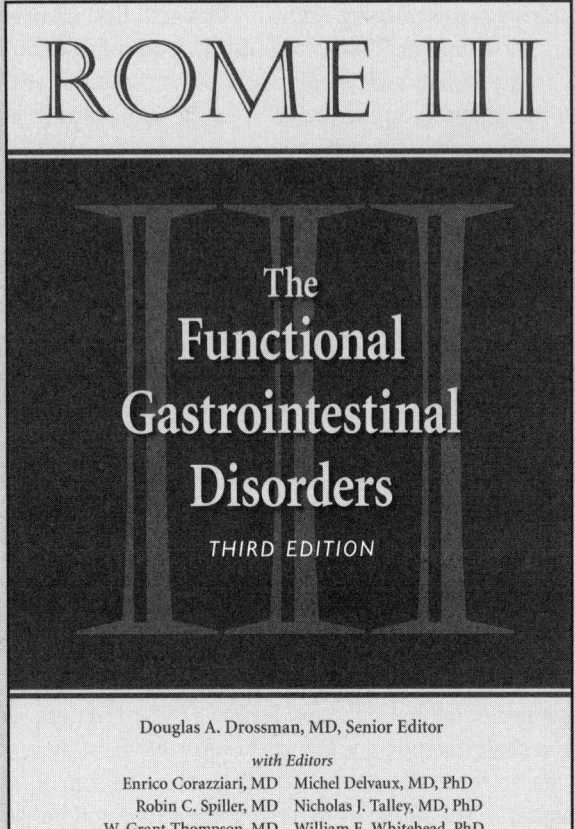

Rome III: The Functional Gastrointestinal Disorders
is the latest and most comprehensive information
that can be found for the evaluation and care of patients
with FGIDs. It serves as a valuable resource to general
and specialist physicians, mental health professionals,
and basic and clinical investigators involved
in the study and care of FGID patients.

You can order *Rome III*
at the Rome Foundation Web site:
www.theromefoundation.org

Acknowledgments

I am grateful to the board of the Rome Foundation for entrusting me with the task of writing this book as an explanatory supplement of *Rome III: The Functional Gastrointestinal Disorders*. Their support has been valuable. Board members Bill Whitehead and John Kellow were among several that assisted me with certain parts of the text. However the lion's share of support and assistance was provided by our senior editor, Doug Drossman, without whom this book could not have been accomplished. Diane Feldman went beyond the call of duty improving my frequent lapses into faulty or unintelligible prose. Jerry Schoendorf's illustrations speak for themselves. As always, my greatest support and inspiration was my wife, Susan. In the end, though, I must accept responsibility for any shortcomings in the book, for which I beg my readers' indulgence.

Dr. Thompson is a consultant with Genpharm ULC, Axcan Pharma, Inc., Procter & Gamble Pharmaceuticals, and Wyeth.

*To
colleagues
from around the world
whose collaboration over many years
made this book possible*

PART 1 About the Functional Gastrointestinal Disorders

Introduction

Part 1 addresses the science upon which our understanding of gut symptoms is based. Chapter 1 explains the functional gastrointestinal disorders (FGIDs). Because it is symptoms that bring patients to their doctors, they must be diagnosed by their symptoms. Using this approach, we have learned a good deal about the nature of these disorders, and the symptoms permit us to classify them into individual syndromes. Chapter 2 explains that the FGIDs are very common throughout the world and that, while never fatal, they can trouble people periodically throughout their lives. Chapter 3 outlines the anatomy and normal functioning of the gastrointestinal tract, the gut's nervous system, and its interaction with the brain. Finally, chapter 4 briefly summarizes what is known about gut malfunctioning and other influences that may be responsible for functional gut symptoms. Many issues must be considered if we are to better understand the disorders. These include abnormalities in the affected person's intestinal physiology, his physical and emotional environment, and his psychological status. These chapters set the stage for part 2, wherein the nature and diagnosis of the individual FGIDS are explained.

1 What Are the Functional Gastrointestinal Disorders?

Introduction

Everyone experiences symptoms occasionally. Some have an obvious cause—pain from a clumsy hammer blow to the thumb, or nausea from a rushed meal. Others, upon investigation, are found to have a medical explanation—abdominal pain due to a peptic ulcer, or faintness due to low blood sugar. Still others have no observable cause. Symptoms that lack a conventional medical explanation are very common. They may be with us from childhood. We usually consider them of little consequence, or part of living. They include such sensations as transient headaches, muscle pains, gut cramps, and numbness of the extremities.

Symptoms are highly personal. They intrude in our private world and are shared with our fellows mainly through words. Our facial grimaces and other nonverbal communication may let others know that we suffer in some way, but they will not know from what we suffer until we tell them. Think of how we must struggle to understand the symptoms of a crying baby. We know when animals suffer too, but because they lack articulation we cannot know the nature of their suffering. Only through language can we understand another's pain. We all understand useful words like *pain, nausea, numbness,* and *bloating,* but *dyspepsia, rumination,* or *esophageal pain* are more obscure and ambiguous. Although we may readily understand the nature of another's reported symptoms, we must rely entirely on their words to learn about severity, location, and provoking factors. These are subject not only to the nature of the injury (if there is one), but also the prior experience, beliefs, and mood of the sufferer. After all, none of us has any basis of comparison. We can say with authority that our pain is better, or worse, or the same, but we have no means of ranking our pain against that of other people.

Sometimes symptoms become chronic, repetitive, and severe. There may be groups of symptoms that suggest a disturbance or *syndrome* in the intestines, the head, the bladder, the reproductive organs, or elsewhere. When these interfere with normal living or seem to warn of a disease, they prompt medical attention and become, at least for the moment, a medical problem. For some

3

chronic conditions, no conventional medical explanation can be found. Such conditions are called *functional disorders,* and those that seem to emanate from the intestines are called the *functional gastrointestinal disorders* (FGIDs). Their defining characteristic is that the manifestly altered functioning of the gut's nerves, muscles, and hormones has no known cause.

For a number of years, teams of experts from around the world have been working to develop a classification and clinical approach for the FGIDs—a group of disorders that afflicts many people but is little understood. The teams report on diagnostic criteria and on the latest medical evidence concerning the recognition and management of FGIDs. Their reports are published in a book that has become a valuable reference for professionals and researchers working with patients who have these disorders. *Rome III: the Functional Gastrointestinal Disorders* is the latest edition of that book. *Understanding the Irritable Gut* is designed to explain the elements of *Rome III* to nonspecialist health professionals and the public. (For more information about *Rome III* and the work of the Rome Foundation, refer to the preface.)

Symptoms and Pathology

It is commonly believed that each symptom has a cause, if only it could be discovered. From ancient times, people ignorant of pathology have invented elaborate explanations for symptoms. Often these encompass the mystical or spiritual. Symptoms might be payment for sin, signal the inexplicable wrath of the gods, or result from a slothful lifestyle. Some societies blame illness on the "evil eye." Systems that have been developed to treat symptoms theorize possible sources; chiropractors attribute symptoms to spinal "subluxation," acupuncturists blame a disturbance of "Qi." Everyone reckons their intestinal symptoms result from "something I ate."

The most important developments in our understanding of disease occurred during the Enlightenment (roughly the eighteenth century), when physicians began to examine the bodies of their patients after death and the science of pathology was born. For example, in the early nineteenth century, physicians examined patients who died of the complications of peptic ulcer disease, and were able to attribute a patient's premortem symptoms to an ulcer they discovered while examining his stomach. As intestinal surgery became common later that century, surgeons could discover pathology in living patients. With such observations, it became possible to predict what a pathologist or surgeon would eventually find by carefully analyzing a patient's symptoms. The characteristic pattern of upper abdominal pain, often occurring predictably at night or after meals and sometimes relieved by eating, helped physicians to diagnose a peptic ulcer without actually seeing it. As knowledge increased, doctors could identify internal illness with a skilled physical examination. A doctor feeling a patient's abdomen might detect an enlarged liver caused by metastatic cancer, or an abdominal mass due to an intestine inflamed by

Crohn's disease. Armed with such knowledge, physicians came to know their patient's enemy and to take steps to correct the underlying defect.

Symptoms without Pathology
("Functional" versus "Organic" Diseases)

Not all symptoms lead to a logical conclusion, however. Many remain unexplained and, as doctors of our generation have learned with dismay, typical symptoms of a peptic ulcer may occur without one being found, even when the stomach and duodenum are examined by endoscopy. This condition has been called "nonulcer" or *functional dyspepsia*. Indeed, all of the FGIDs are characterized by intestinal symptoms that may, at first hearing, suggest a structural disease of the gut, but upon closer examination none is discovered. That is, the underlying determinants of the disorders are not explained by structural damage to the intestines. Rather they are understood as abnormalities in the functioning (i.e., physiology) of the gut. These disturbed functions may involve intestinal movements (motility), intestinal nerve sensitivity, secretions into the intestines, or the activities of nerves and chemicals (neuropeptides) that control these functions. The intestinal tract is believed to cause symptoms by functioning abnormally. Despite this assumption, it has proven very difficult to distinguish normal from abnormal. Moreover, observed abnormalities of gut dysmotility may be epiphenomena; that is, they may exist with the symptoms only through coincidence, not as a cause. Even when such symptoms are weakly correlated to a gut disturbance, it is far from certain what causes the disturbance itself. For example, in functional constipation even a measurably slow intestinal transit is unexplained.

Symptoms without a clear cause pose a dilemma for physicians and patients alike. Doctors are trained to believe that symptoms imply a discoverable abnormality. If they can find the abnormality, they can repair it and eliminate the symptoms. Hence, in a patient with pain in the upper abdomen, a physician examining the inside of the stomach with an endoscope may discover an ulcer. Then by prescribing appropriate drug therapy the physician can not only heal that ulcer, but prevent its recurrence. However, the situation is quite different when no ulcer is found and further examination fails to turn up any abnormality, or when a discovered ulcer is treated and the pain remains. Treatments become far less straightforward and cure of the symptoms less tangible. In the former case there is a potentially life-threatening "organic" disease that lends itself to prompt diagnosis and successful treatment. In the latter instance, the disorder is said to be "functional"—no life-threatening "organic" explanation exists, and no treatment is completely effective.

Disease and Illness

We must distinguish disease from illness. Disease is what a pathologist, clinician, or any trained physician can observe. It may be a peptic ulcer, seen as

Structural and "Functional" Disease

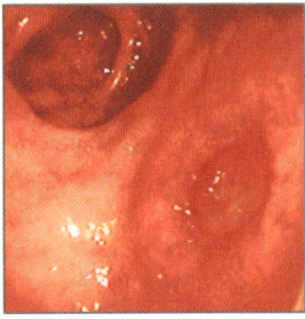
Peptic ulcer

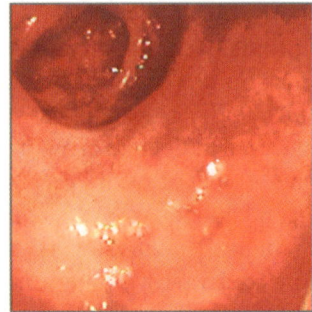
Non-ulcer dyspepsia

Figure 1-1. The photo on the left shows an endoscopic view of a peptic ulcer in the duodenum of a patient who had typical meal-related and nocturnal upper abdominal pain. The view on the right shows no pathology in a patient with similar symptoms. Such a patient is said to have "nonulcer" or "functional" dyspepsia. (*Photos by author*)

a crater in the lining of the stomach or duodenum (figure 1-1), or diabetes, signified by high blood-sugar test results. In such cases, the patient's symptoms are seen to be "legitimized" by the presence of a tangible cause, and treatment can be logical and precise. Illness, on the other hand is what one feels. It may or may not accompany a known disease, but the patient feels ill, and at that moment cares little for the nature of his disease or its cause. If one is able to cure the underlying disease by administering treatment, the symptoms usually improve. However, what if there is illness without disease? A person with a functional disorder has illness with an array of possible causes that are not readily observed to explain it, and will probably be disappointed to discover that no specific treatment is available. Nevertheless, we shall see that, despite the lack of specific therapy for the FGIDs, there are measures that can help.

The Biopsychosocial Model

As noted, the distinction between disease and illness is imprecise. One can have a disease without symptoms; that is, a disease without illness. An example is a silent (asymptomatic) peptic ulcer that is found only by accident during tests or surgery for some other purpose. Sometimes, cure of a disease may not eliminate all symptoms, suggesting that the illness has a functional as well as an organic component. When we label a patient's illness as "functional," it does not mean that a specific organic finding does not exist; it may later become clear through repeated examination or better technology that there is a cause after all. Then, the "functional" symptoms may be explained by "organic" findings. "Functional" becomes "organic." Among those who have symptoms with no evident disease there often remains the hope that a treatable disease exists, if only doctors knew how to recognize it. The perceived failure to identify a cause requires careful explanation if the patient's response to treatment is not to be marred by frustration.

In the first chapter of the *Rome III* book, Drossman recalls the separation of mind and body or "dualism" that characterized the philosophy of the Enlightenment philosopher René Descartes. Such separation permitted the conduct of postmortem examination after the soul had departed, and the subsequent scientific advances described above. But, given the times, there was no way to explain symptoms without pathology and, with no explanation, the patient was thought to have a psychiatric condition or be "possessed." Drossman describes the overweening tendency to attribute all illness to specific diseases as "reductionism." As a result of that tendency, some physicians and the public may stigmatize all illnesses that we are unable to adequately explain as mental illnesses.

Reductionism has served medical science well. In designing an experiment addressing a single question, such as the potential cause of a disease, it is necessary to employ controls. That is, all other factors that might influence the disease are held constant during the experiment lest they bias the result (see chapter 15). In such an experiment, the result is reduced to the answer to a single question. Nevertheless, Drossman is correct; our ignorance and insistence upon a single all-encompassing explanation tempts us to categorize unexplained illnesses in a lower order. Reductionism, however useful it may be to science, is an unsuitable basis for the management of an individual's illness.

Another view is that the causation of illness—and to some extent disease itself—is multifactorial; that is, in an individual it is seldom attributable to a single phenomenon. In the *biopsychosocial model* of disease, illustrated in figure 1-2, a host of factors—genetic, environmental, psychosocial, physiological, and pathological—interact to produce the symptoms and behaviors that we know as illness. (Internist and psychoanalyst George Engel originated the term "biopsychosocial model.") Even where the pathology is overt, as with an ulcer, one person may be disabled by pain while another may report no symptoms. Adolescents respond to their acne in a social and psychological as well as biological manner. It is probable that no human illness manifests itself in solely pathological terms.

This model is particularly suited to the study and management of functional disorders. For the scientist who must work with reductionist models, the ideas in figure 1-2 force an open mind. We can make no assumptions about the cause(s) of irritable bowel syndrome or dyspepsia despite the passionately promoted theories to be discussed in chapter 4. For a century peptic ulcer was thought to be due to excessive stomach acid secretion. This belief led to sur-

8 Understanding the Irritable Gut

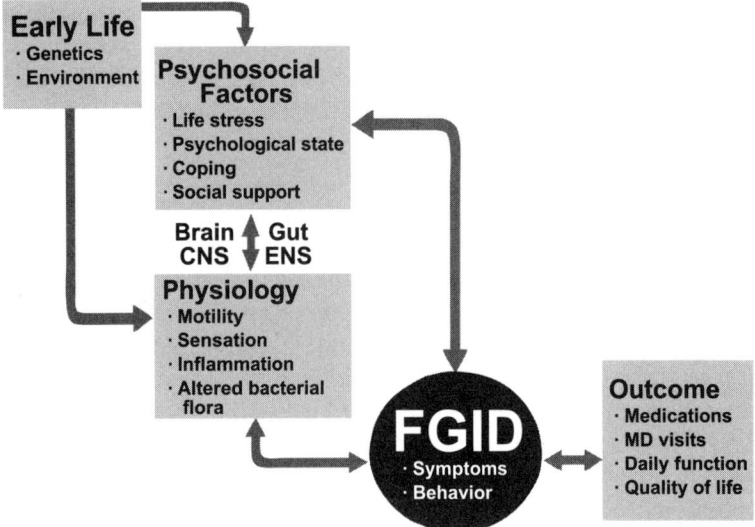

Figure 1-2. A biopsychosocial conceptualization of the pathogenesis and clinical expression of the functional gastrointestinal disorders. This model portrays the relationships between psychosocial and physiological phenomena, functional gastrointestinal symptoms, and clinical outcome. CNS = central nervous system, ENS = enteric nervous system. (Adapted from *Rome III: the Functional Gastrointestinal Disorders*, p. 4.)

gical and medical treatments that were designed to decrease the stomach's acid production. Such was the rigidity of prevailing opinion that in the 1980s, when Marshall and Warren discovered that bacteria called *Helicobacter pylori* caused ulcers, the truth was disbelieved for years. The biopsychosocial model embraces all possible contributing factors—a broader vision that should permit no such blinkered view of the FGIDs.

The model also has important lessons for the clinician and the patient. While no one cause can be identified, the many factors that manifestly influence the course of an individual's illness can be constructively addressed. These include diagnosis, diet, life situations, and other manageable factors that are discussed in part 3 of this book. Because symptoms constitute the illness, treatment should aspire to relieve them and to make the sufferer feel better about them. Satisfying this aspiration calls as much upon the "art" as the science of medicine.

The Functional Gastrointestinal Disorders

Not so long ago, the FGIDs lacked definition. The diagnosis was usually arrived at after exhaustive, expensive, and sometimes dangerous testing had failed to disclose an organic disease. This led the identification of the irritable bowel syndrome (IBS) and other functional gut disorders to be reluctantly and sometimes pejoratively considered "diagnoses of exclusion." Physicians graduated from medical school and postgraduate programs with little understanding of the functional disorders, since few such cases were encountered in the hospitals where they studied. Those patients who were admitted were clinically frustrating and too often became the responsibility of the most junior person on the team. They were "problem patients" who defied rational diagnosis, despite advanced technology, and responded poorly to treatment offered by doctors who often ignored the biopsychosocial nature of their patients' illnesses.

Lack of precise description of these disorders has other consequences. In 1988, Klein complained that patients entered in clinical trials were improperly described, so that no one could judge to which patients the results might be appropriate. With no agreed-upon diagnosis, it is neither possible to select suitable subjects for clinical trials, nor subsequently to identify those patients to whom the trial results might apply.

The Rome process that is described in the foreward to this book seeks to change old attitudes and clarify the FGIDs. The various syndromes are classified by presumed anatomical location. (See table 1-1.) Note that a *symptom* is singular, like abdominal pain or diarrhea, while a *syndrome* is a total experience that may include several symptoms. Sometimes in organic diseases, but not in functional disorders, a syndrome might include a physical sign, a certain blood result, or a physiologic measurement. The Rome working teams define the functional gut syndromes, and develop symptom-based diagnostic criteria for each of them through consensus and a peer-review process. The *Rome III* criteria are presented in Appendix A and discussed in the context of individual disorders in part 2 of this book.

As specific explanations are discovered for these disorders, one by one they may be dropped from the list and no longer regarded as functional. Some dream of the day when we can confidently identify the cause of each of the disorders, and eventually through effective treatment eliminate them from the human experience. Others feel that functional illnesses are so influenced by one's environment, psyche, attitude, and other items indicated in figure 1-2, that they will always be a challenge. Indeed they seem part of the human condition, leading William Osler a century ago to admonish physicians, " . . . to cure sometimes, to relieve often, to comfort always."

Conclusion

Illness consists of the symptoms we experience. They may or may not result from a specific pathology or physiologic abnormality. If they do, they are labeled "organic," and if not, "functional." These last two terms satisfy very few experts. "Organic" invites concentration on discovery of pathology and denial

Table 1-1. The Functional Gastrointestinal Disorders

A. Functional Esophageal Disorders
    A1. Functional heartburn
    A2. Functional chest pain of presumed esophageal origin
    A3. Functional dysphagia
    A4. Globus

B. Functional Gastroduodenal Disorders
    B1. Functional dyspepsia
        B1a. Postprandial distress syndrome (PDS)
        B1b. Epigastric pain syndrome (EPS)
    B2. Belching disorders
        B2a. Aerophagia
        B2b. Unspecified excessive belching
    B3. Nausea and vomiting disorders
        B3c. Chronic idiopathic vomiting (CIN)
        B3b. Functional vomiting
        B3c. Cyclic vomiting syndrome (CVS)
    B4. Rumination syndrome in adults

C. Functional Bowel Disorders
    C1. Irritable bowel syndrome (IBS)
    C2. Functional bloating
    C3. Functional constipation
    C4. Functional diarrhea
    C5. Unspecified functional bowel disorder

D. Functional Abdominal Pain Syndrome (FAPS)

E. Functional Gallbladder and Sphincter of Oddi (SO) Disorders
    E1. Functional gallbladder disorder
    E2. Functional biliary SO disorder
    E3. Functional pancreatic SO disorder

F. Functional Anorectal Disorders
    F1. Functional fecal incontinence
    F2. Functional anorectal pain
        F2a. Chronic proctalgia
            F2a1. Levator ani syndrome
            F2a2. Unspecified functional anorectal pain
        F2b. Proctalgia fugax
    F3. Functional defecation disorders
        F3a. Dyssynergic defecation
        F3b. Inadequate defecatory propulsion

Adapted from *Rome III: the Functional Gastrointestinal Disorders*, p. 6.

of the biopsychosocial model. However, one cannot contemplate pathology without understanding illness. "Functional" implies disturbed function—in this case gastrointestinal function—but ignores the psychosocial situation and personal experience of someone experiencing the symptoms. Moreover, for some, "functional" came to mean insoluble, and sometimes seemed pejorative. Nevertheless, the best-informed minds can agree upon no better terms, so we must accept "organic" and "functional" for now, remembering that there is nothing pejorative about illness, however experienced.

Sources

Creed F, Levy RL, Bradley LA, Drossman DA, Francisconi C, Naliboff BD, Olden KW. Psychosocial aspects of the functional gastrointestinal disorders. In: Drossman DA, Corazziari E, Delvaux M, Spiller RC, Talley NJ, Thompson WG, Whitehead WE, eds. *Rome III: The Functional Gastrointestinal Disorders*. McLean, VA: Degnon Associates, Inc.; 2006:295-267.

Drossman, DA. Presidential Address: Gastrointestinal Illness and Biopsychosocial Model. *Psychosomatic Medicine*. 1998;60(3):258-267.

Drossman DA. The functional gastrointestinal disorders and the *Rome III* process. In: Drossman DA, Corazziari E, Delvaux M, Spiller RC, Talley NJ, Thompson WG, Whitehead WE, eds. *Rome III: The Functional Gastrointestinal Disorders*. McLean, VA: Degnon Associates Inc.; 2006:1-30.

Klein KB. Controlled treatment trials in the irritable bowel syndrome: a critique. *Gastroenterology*. 1988;95:232-241.

Toner BB, Chang L, Fukudo S, Guthrie E, Locke GR, Norton N, Sperber AD. Gender, age, society, culture, and the patient's perspective. In: Drossman DA, Corazziari E, Delvaux M, Spiller RC, Talley NJ, Thompson WG, Whitehead WE, Spiller RC, Talley NJ, Thompson WG, Whitehead WE, eds. *Rome III: The Functional Gastrointestinal Disorders*. McLean, VA: Degnon Associates, Inc.; 2006: 231-293.

2 How Common Are the Functional Gastrointestinal Disorders?

Introduction

Epidemiology is the study of the occurrence in populations of a range of conditions that affect health. When diagnostic criteria for the diagnosis of the functional gastrointestinal disorders (FGIDs) became available, it became possible to survey populations to determine their epidemiology. This chapter briefly describes how the epidemiologic data are acquired and what they mean.

Incidence and Prevalence

Incidence is the "attack rate" of a disease. That is, it is the number of *new* cases of a disease, disorder, or other medical state that develop in a defined population within a certain period, say one year. Prevalence is the number of people with the condition within the same population *at any one time*, say now, or within six months or a year. Because the FGIDs are usually chronic, recurring, and often life-long, the discussion here will deal solely with prevalence, principally the one-year prevalence.

How Prevalence is Determined

To recognize a disease in a given population, investigators must employ a generally agreed-upon and reproducible "biomarker" of that disease and apply it to a suitable sample of that population. In the case of physical or "organic" disorders, this may mean a physical measurement. Examples might be blood pressure, body weight, or blood sugar, with predetermined cutoff values that identify an abnormal trait. Cancer cases might be identified by biopsy and coronary artery disease by electrocardiogram changes during chest pain. In the case of the FGIDs, there are no such generally agreed-upon and reproducible biomarkers. Because they are manifest only by symptoms, it is by symptoms that they must be identified. Hence, diagnostic criteria for the FGIDs were developed, first by independent researchers and, since 1988, through the Rome process. (See the preface to this book to learn more about the Rome process.) It is upon such symptom criteria that a survey's questions are based.

However, it is one thing for experts to identify the features of a disorder such as the irritable bowel syndrome (IBS), but quite another to design the questions to be uniformly presented to the respondents without risk of bias. Faulty questionnaires lead to faulty data. How a question is asked can greatly influence the answer. For example, few would answer "no" to the question, "Have you ever had abdominal pain?" However, if the frequency, severity, location, and time period are specified, the question should capture only those with more important or relevant pain. The *Rome II* and *Rome III* books provide questionnaires to set standards for future surveys and to assist researchers who recruit subjects for clinical trials and other research.

A most critical issue in any survey is how well the interviewed subjects represent the population they are purported to represent. An inappropriate sample may not be representative, which could lead to faulty or biased information about the larger population.

The Prevalence of the FGIDs
Historical Note

In collaboration with K.W. Heaton in 1978, I conducted the first survey of nonpatients (mainly health care workers, sailors, and retirees) that sought to determine the prevalence of functional gut symptoms in apparently healthy people. We used among other instruments the Manning criteria that were previously developed by Heaton's team, and found to our surprise that IBS as well as many other FGIDs, from globus to proctalgia fugax, were very common in this population. Soon thereafter, Drossman produced similar data in a U.S. population. After the *Rome I* criteria became available, Drossman conducted a survey of a large, commercially collected sample of people throughout the United States. That survey confirmed that the Rome-defined symptoms and syndromes were common in that population as well. Since then, there have been myriad studies around the world demonstrating similar prevalences. Figures 2-1 and 2-2 show these global prevalence data for dyspepsia and IBS, based upon surveys that, for the most part, employed *Rome I* criteria.

FGID Prevalence

Despite small quantitative differences between the many FGID surveys throughout the world, the data confirm the great prevalence of many functional gut disorders. Prevalence differences in men and women and in the individual disorders may be attributable to culture and language variations, evolving criteria, and the variable nature and quality of the survey questionnaires. Table 2-1 presents the results of the only FGID survey to date that used the *Rome II* criteria. Sixty-two percent of people experienced Rome-defined FGIDs.

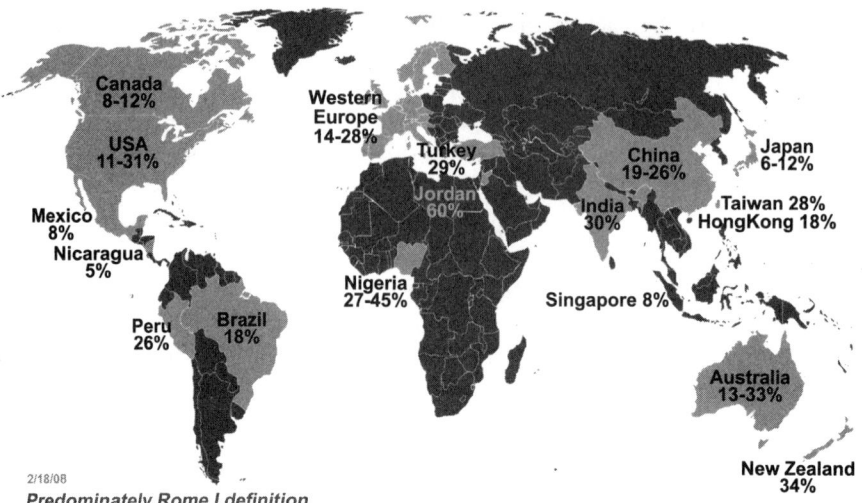

Figure 2-1. Worldwide prevalence of dyspepsia. These data are from surveys that mainly used *Rome I* criteria. The data are dependent upon the criteria, the population chosen for the survey, the design of the questions, and how the questions are asked.

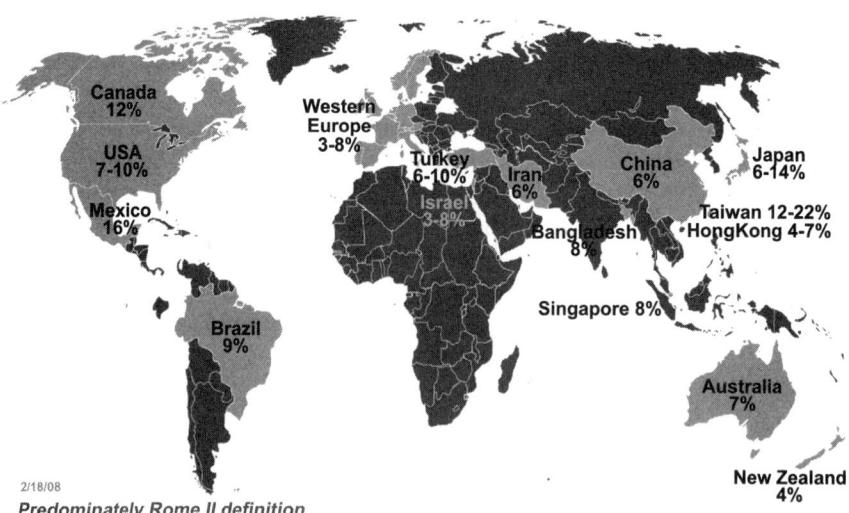

Figure 2-2. Worldwide prevalence of the irritable bowel syndrome. Most of the data are from surveys that used *Rome I* or *Rome II* criteria. The varying prevalences are due in part to differences in culture, language, and IBS criteria chosen, but also to the nature or manner of administration of the questionnaire.

Table 2-1. Prevalence of the Individual Functional Gastrointestinal Disorders Using *Rome II* Classification and Questionnaire

Functional Gastrointestinal Disorders	N	All (Total = 1149) %	Males (556) %	Females (593) %
A. Esophageal disorders				
A1. Globus	29	2.5	2.5	2.5
A2. Rumination	9	0.8	1.1	0.5
A3. Functional chest pain	23	2.0	1.7	2.2
A4. Functional heartburn	256	22.3	24.6	20.2
A5. Functional dysphagia	25	2.2	1.8	2.6
B. Gastroduodenal disorders				
B1. Functional dyspepsia	21	1.8	0.9	2.6
B1a. Ulcer-like	10	0.9	0.1	1.6*
B2b. Dysmotility-like	10	0.9	0.8	1.0
B2. Aerophagia	112	9.7	11.3	8.3
B3. Functional vomiting	5	0.4	0.4	0.4
C. Bowel disorders				
C1. Irritable bowel syndrome	139	12.1	8.7	15.2*
C1a. Diarrhea-predominant	0	0.0	0.0	0.0
C1b. Constipation-predominant	55	4.8	2.8	6.7*
C2. Functional abdominal bloating	151	13.1	8.5	17.5*
C3. Functional constipation	241	21.0	15.6	26.1*
C4. Functional diarrhea	98	8.5	9.8	7.2
D. Functional abdominal pain				
D1. Functional abdominal pain syndrome	6	0.5	0.5	0.5
D2. Unspecified functional abdominal pain	24	2.1	1.4	2.8
E. Biliary disorders				
E1. Gallbladder dysfunction	0	0.0	0.0	0.0
E2. Sphincter of Oddi dysfunction	0	0.0	0.0	0.0
F. Anorectal disorders				
F1. Functional incontinence	79	6.9	4.8	8.9*
F1a. Soiling	60	5.2	3.8	6.6*
F1b. Gross incontinence	18	1.6	0.9	2.2
F2. Functional anorectal pain	193	16.8	16.4	17.1
F2a. Levator ani syndrome	28	2.4	2.5	2.4
F2b. Proctalgia fugax	53	4.6	3.4	5.6
F3. Pelvic floor dyssynergia	0	0.0	0.0	0.0
Any FGID	701	61.7	57.6	65.6*

*Statistical difference between men and women
Adapted from Thompson et al, 2002, p. 228

16 Understanding the Irritable Gut

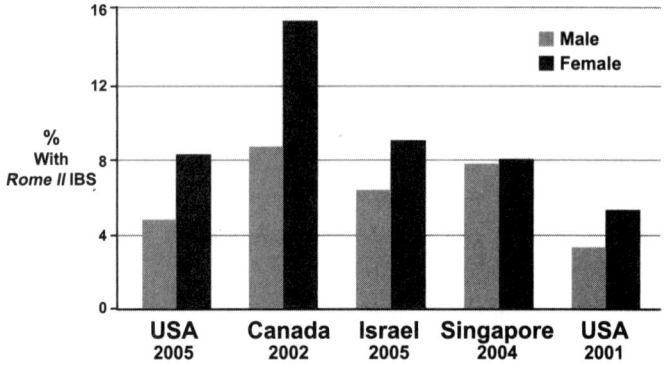

Figure 2-3. Gender differences in the irritable bowel syndrome in several countries. The predominance in females among those with irritable bowel syndrome in the West often is not found in Asian surveys.

The IBS occurs in 10% to 20% of the adult population. In most of the world, IBS is twice as common in women as men, but in certain Asian communities, the gender ratio may be even or reversed (see figure 2-3). IBS is also common in children. The FGIDs begin in youth and recur periodically for many years, even a lifetime. Through sequential surveys of the same population, Talley and colleagues determined that IBS occurred in about 18% of their study population, but there was a somewhat different group of affected individuals in each survey. Thus, at least some people acquire and lose IBS characteristics as the years pass.

More detailed discussions of FGID prevalence appear in chapters 7 through 12 of the *Rome III* book. These data cannot be interpreted without consideration of the methodological limitations of the surveys and a perspective of the disorders' severity and social cost.

Limitations of the Data

To date, none of the FGID surveys has been conducted in a true random sample of the population. Therefore, one can apply the data to a population of a country or an ethnic group only in a general way. Certainly patients or hospital employees cannot be considered representative of all people. A survey of volunteers is suspect, as they may have a special interest in the topic, and are somewhat likely to have an FGID. Few reports discuss the randomness of their subjects' selection. Nevertheless, the message from the data collected so far is that the FGIDs are common, no matter what the sample. Therefore, this limitation is a relative one.

Other limitations are the criteria by which affected persons are identified and the quality of the questionnaire used to gather the data. These alone could be the subject of a chapter, but suffice it here to mention three things. First, survey answers rely on the patient's memory and his or her interpretation of the importance of the questions. After three months one's memory of symptoms begins to fade. Second, criteria drawn up by consensus among doctors who see patients may not be valid for the general public. And third, how the questions are asked may determine the answer, especially if the subject feels the interviewer would welcome a positive answer.

As a result, the data provide an imperfect idea of how common or important gut sensations are in the population. No questionnaire can accurately assess severity. As discussed in the last chapter, symptoms are a private matter. Their expression as an illness might signal their importance, but an anonymously administered questionnaire can only provide hints. According to every survey in which it was asked, fewer than half of those with IBS had sought medical attention for it. These individuals must consider their symptoms to be mild or unimportant.

An Epidemiologic Perspective of the FGIDs

Not all patients who are identified by questionnaire to have an FGID such as IBS are ill, and still fewer are patients. Here is a problem. Much of the available IBS data is derived from studies of the most severely affected patients who may constitute as few as 1% of the whole (see figure 2-4). Therefore, advice to a patient attending a specialty clinic may be inappropriate for someone in primary care. Moreover, no interpretation of the data should persuade us that uncomplaining people with FGIDs need medical care.

There is a further hierarchy among those who do see doctors (see figure 2-5). Most are cared for in primary care by a general practitioner, family doctor, or internist. Many of these patients are mildly affected and are concerned that they may have cancer. They want to know what the symptoms mean and what should be done about them. More severely affected patients may return with continuing symptoms and seek relief. The most seriously affected patients are often troubled and dependent, and often consult FGID experts at tertiary care centers. Most research occurs in such highly specialized places.

People affected by an organic disease such as diabetes eventually seek medical care. Treatment guidelines as to diet, medication, and insulin are well established by research and are universal—they apply equally to most similar medical care situations in developed countries. This is simply not the case in the FGIDs. The degree to which a person with a functional disease is affected depends upon many things: the difficult-to-assess severity of the symptoms, the degree to which they interfere with daily living, the individual's mood and psychosocial situation, the options available in his community or jurisdiction for the care of that disorder, and the success of a primary physician's diagnosis, reassurance, and advice.

IBS: A World View

14% of adults have IBS

30% see primary care doctor

Primary care
20% referred to gastroenterologist

Secondary care 6%

Tertiary care
Patients studied in academic centers: ~1%

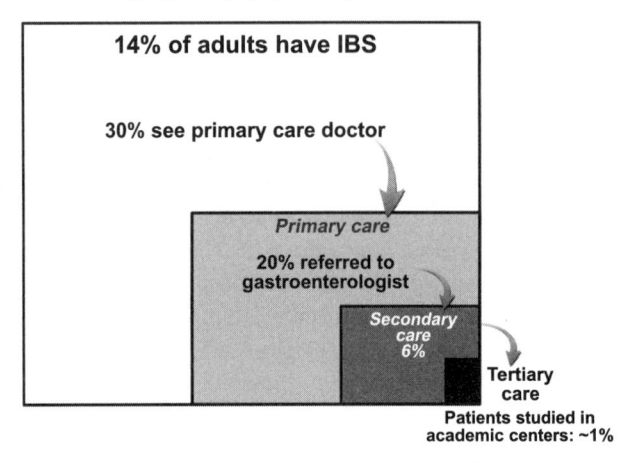

Figure 2-4. A perspective. The prevalence of the irritable bowel syndrome may be 14%, but only about 30% of those affected see a primary care doctor. Of these, about 20% are referred to specialists. Fewer still are referred to academic centers where most physiological, psychological, and treatment studies are done. Data from such studies may not be applicable to patients in primary care, nor to those who do not consult a physician.

Severity

- Dependent and coping ineffectively
- Impaired employment and social functioning
- Physical and psychosocial co-morbidity

Severe

- Persistent symptoms and stress
- Impaired quality of life
- Seeks relief

Moderate

- What do symptoms mean?
- Worried about cancer
- What should be done?

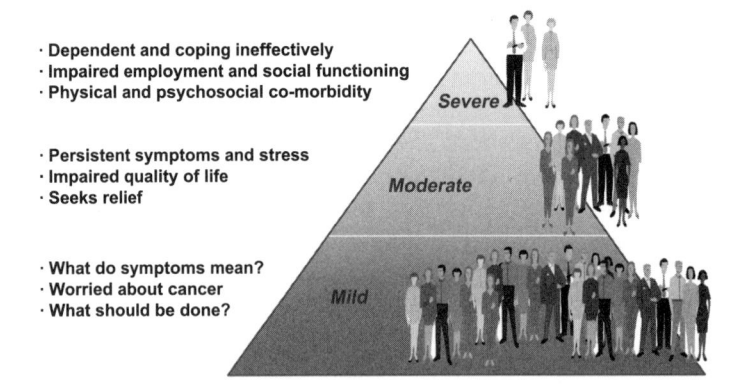

Mild

Figure 2-5. There is a hierarchy among IBS patients that is correlated with symptom severity. Patients with the mildest symptoms are found mainly in primary care; they are concerned with the meaning and implication of their symptoms. The more severe the patients' symptoms, the more likely they are to be referred to and given treatment by specialists, and the more complicated their management.

Conclusion

Despite their limitations, population surveys teach us that the FGIDs are very common all over the world. However, it appears that most of those people identified with these disorders do not consider themselves ill, and do not consult physicians. Unlike cancer or heart disease, there seems to be no reason to urge such people to seek care. No cure is available, and if they are managing nicely there is no evidence that seeking them out for such care would be beneficial to them. It might increase doctors' workloads and shorten their time with those whose symptoms have compelled them to consult a physician. Among those people who do see doctors there is a further hierarchy based on how severely the symptoms affect the patient. Careful consideration of the patient's quality of life, his psychosocial situation, and the available treatment options should help a physician to advise a personalized program of medical care.

Sources

Drossman DA, Li Z, Andruzzi E, et al. U.S. householder survey of functional gastrointestinal disorders: prevalence, sociodemography and health impact. *Dig Dis Sci*. 1993;38:1569-1580.

Manning AP, Thompson WG, Heaton KW, Morris AF. Towards positive diagnosis of the irritable bowel. *Br Med J*. 1978;2:653-654.

Talley NJ, Weaver AL, Zinsmeister AR, Melton LJ. Onset and disappearance of gastrointestinal symptoms and functional gastrointestinal disorders. *Am J Epidemiol*. 1992;136:165-177.

Thompson WG, Heaton KW. Functional bowel disorders in apparently healthy people. *Gastroenterology*. 1980;79:283-288.

Thompson WG, Irvine EJ, Pare P, Ferrazzi S, Rance L. Functional gastrointestinal disorders in Canada: first population based survey using the Rome II criteria with suggestions for improving the questionnaire. *Dig Dis Sci*. 2002;47:225-235.

3 The Gut: How It Works

Introduction

This chapter contains a brief overview of the anatomy and physiology (normal functioning) of the gut. The purpose is to set the stage for later chapters where the possible causes of the functional gastrointestinal disorders (FGIDs) are described. The anatomic and physiologic descriptions progress according to the anatomic regions where the disorders that are listed in the *Rome III* classification are believed to originate (see table 1-1). Next, under "Neurogastroenterology," is a discussion of the nerves and chemicals that govern gut function in a "gut brain" called the *enteric nervous system*. There follows a discussion of the brain-gut interactions that have a very prominent role in the FGIDs, and the chapter ends with a brief description of gastrointestinal motility.

Anatomy and Function

The Esophagus

The esophagus is a twenty-centimeter-long muscular tube stretching from the throat to where it enters the stomach behind the lower end of the breastbone. It is an active organ, responding to a swallow with a pressure wave (peristalsis) that moves the swallowed material towards the stomach. Its activities include gatekeeping by two valves or sphincters—one at either end of the organ. These sphincters consist of segments of muscular contraction that must relax for food to proceed. The *upper esophageal sphincter* opens with a swallow and is therefore voluntary. Some believe that dysfunction here accounts for the globus sensation.

The *lower esophageal sphincter* (LES) not only must relax to allow food to enter the stomach, but it must remain closed between swallows to prevent stomach acid and food from refluxing back into the unprotected esophagus. Reflux occurs when the stomach's internal pressure exceeds that of the esophagus, and the LES cannot retain acid gastric contents in the stomach. The most common symptom due to reflux is a burning chest sensation known as heartburn. This often occurs when one bends over or lies down after a meal. A similar symptom that occurs in some people who have no demonstrable acid reflux

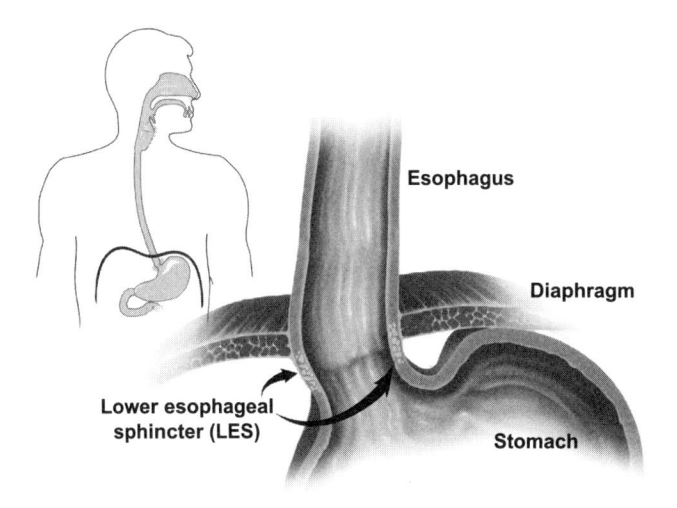

Figure 3-1. The lower esophagus.

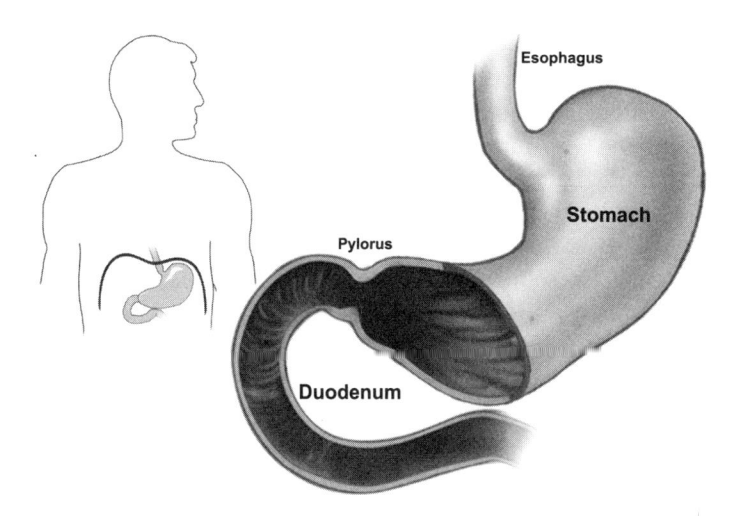

Figure 3-2. The gastroduodenum ("gastro" means stomach).

is known as functional heartburn. Several other functional esophageal disorders are believed to be due to a malfunctioning LES and lower esophagus.

The Gastroduodenum

The *stomach* is the receptacle in which swallowed food is collected. Normally collapsed, it must relax to accommodate a meal. The stomach is a very active organ; vigorous contractions of its muscular coat grind up food and eventually force it through a narrow muscular valve known as the *pylorus*. Immediately beyond the pylorus is a curved segment of small intestine called the *duodenum*. The stomach and duodenum are considered together here, since many diseases such as peptic ulcer occur in both organs. Dyspepsia is believed to originate in the *gastroduodenum* (the stomach and the duodenum).

Within the wall of the stomach are cells specialized to produce very strong acid that is capable of reducing the stomach contents' pH to as low as 2 (neutral is 7). Acid assists the initial steps of digestion and activates enzymes that begin to digest food constituents. Excess stomach acid was long believed to cause peptic ulcers in the stomach and duodenum. During the twentieth century great effort was expended to reduce gastric acid production through medical and surgical means. In the early 1990s it became clear that an inflamed stomach lining (gastritis) and peptic ulcers were caused by long ignored bacteria that infect the lining of the stomach, now called *Helicobacter pylori*. It took some years before physicians realized that they could kill this organism with antibiotics and cure peptic ulcers once and for all. Thereafter, peptic ulcer became a much less threatening, and less common, disease. Nevertheless, many people continue to suffer from dyspepsia. Dysfunctioning gastroduodenal motility, excess acid secretion, and/or *H. pylori* infection are blamed.

The Intestines

Intestine and *bowel* may be used interchangeably. There is a large intestine and a small intestine; the large intestine is commonly called the *colon*. To further confuse the terminology, these are also referred to as the large *gut* and the small *gut*. The small intestine is a muscular organ whose length varies considerably, depending upon the state of contraction of its two muscle coats. The muscle here is called *smooth muscle* and is under autonomic control, unlike skeletal muscle which we voluntarily contract or relax. The small intestine's principal function is to digest food and then absorb nutrients from the products of digestion, such as amino acids, fatty acids, and sugars. The first part of the small intestine, the *duodenum* (mentioned above as part of the gastroduodenum), is followed by the *jejunum* and the *ileum*.

The three segments of the small intestine are similar in appearance, but differ in function. The duodenum is the primary site of digestion, assisted by bile and pancreatic enzymes that empty into it from the bile and pancreatic ducts. (See "The Pancreatic and Biliary Systems" below). Most nutrient absorption occurs through the lining of the jejunum, while the ileum is the sole site of vitamin B_{12} absorption and reabsorption of bile salts. Enzymes responsible for the final stages of digestion are situated on the jejunum's internal surface. Examples are disaccharidases, the enzymes that are responsible for the digestion of unabsorbable disaccharides, such as the milk sugar lactose. The products of lactose digestion are the absorbable monosaccharide sugars glucose and galactose.

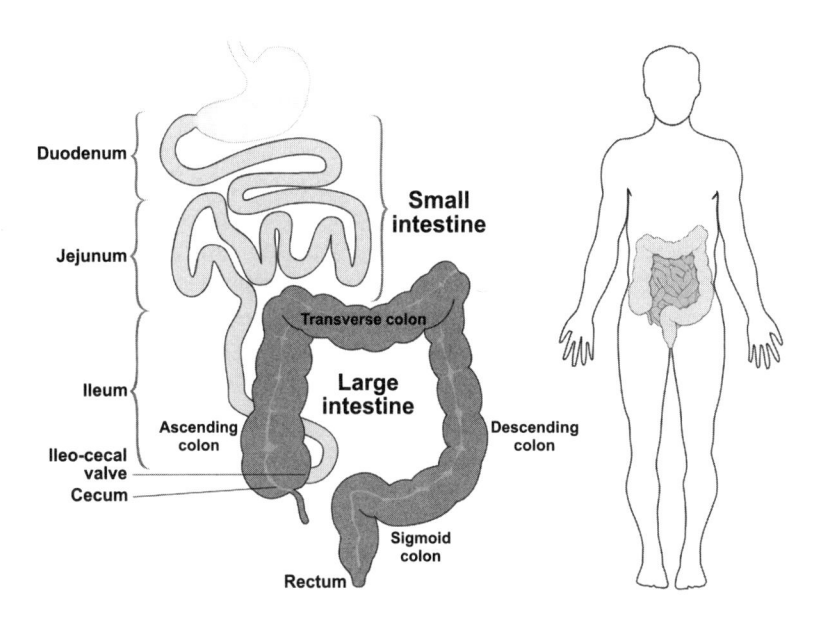

Figure 3-3. The intestines. On the left, the small intestine has been stretched out to show its parts and where it begins and ends. The relative positions of the small and large intestines are shown on the right.

There is a vast flow of water between the intestinal lumen and the rich blood vessel network that surrounds the small intestine. This water exchange in and out of the intestine is approximately eight liters daily (two U.S. gallons). The net volume of water that eventually makes it through the ileocecal valve into the large intestine depends upon many factors, including fluid intake, the body's hydration and mineral balance, bile and intestinal secretion, absorption efficiency, and the speed of intestinal transit. Only a few ounces of fluid eventually get excreted in the stool. This water exchange is finely balanced and important because relatively small changes in secretion or absorption can result in diarrhea or constipation. The bacterial toxin of cholera bacteria causes severe, dehydrating, and potentially lethal diarrhea by causing the small intestine to secrete far more fluid than it is able to absorb.

The small intestine ends at the *ileocecal valve*, a muscular sphincter through which the intestinal content, less most nutrients, flows into the *cecum,* the nearest part of the colon (large intestine). Fluid contents are further mixed there and proceed along the *ascending* and *transverse* segments of the colon, from which more water is slowly absorbed. The remaining soft, solid material is eventually propelled along the *descending* and *sigmoid* segments of the colon and through the *anorectum* as stool. Colon water absorption amounts to about one liter daily and can be altered by laxatives, antidiarrhea drugs, and substances such as bile salts and lactose that in certain diseases may fail to be absorbed in the small intestine.

The small intestine contains few bacteria until it approaches the ileocecal valve. However the contents of the colon are predominantly bacteria and water. There are ten trillion cells in the human body and an estimated ten times that number of individual bacteria in the intestines. These colonic tenants of ours are diverse both in species and in function. Some of them metabolize nutrients without needing oxygen; these are said to be anaerobic. Colonic bacteria usually live in peace with us as their hosts and are responsible for useful and not-so-useful immunologic and metabolic functions. They are capable of metabolizing unabsorbed materials that survive the small intestine, thereby producing energy-rich short-chain fatty acids. In addition, they are responsible for the production of most colonic gases, notably carbon dioxide, hydrogen, and in some cases methane. These bacteria are essential to our health, having made peace with our intestinal immune defenses. However, they can be overcome by hostile bacteria that can cause infectious diarrhea. It is possible that a bacterial infection or changes in the bacterial flora may cause or trigger an irritable bowel.

The large and small intestines are believed to be the site of the functional bowel disorders. However, attempts to identify the precise intestinal malfunction(s) underlying these disorders have so far failed.

The Pancreatic and Biliary Systems

Figure 3-4 shows the *gallbladder* and *pancreas*. Their respective ducts conduct the products of these organs to the duodenum at a point shortly beyond the pylorus. The gallbladder stores bile produced in the liver and discharges it through the bile duct into the duodenum after a meal, particularly a fatty one. Bile contains bile salts that assist in the absorption of fat. These in turn are mostly reabsorbed in the ileum and re-excreted in the liver. Bile also contains the end products of the normal breakdown of the red pigment in aging red blood cells called hemoglobin. These waste pigments are collectively known as bilirubin and account for the brown color of stool. The pancreatic duct conveys enzymes capable of digesting ingested fat, protein, and carbohydrates into their constituent fatty acids, amino acids, and sugars. These components are subsequently absorbed in the jejunum.

Of particular interest in the FGIDs is the *sphincter of Oddi*, the muscular valve located where the bile ducts enter the duodenum. In some individuals, the pancreatic duct shares this sphincter with the bile ducts; in others it has its own sphincter. When the ducts become obstructed with gallstones, severe pain may occur, and the gallbladder and/or pancreas may become acutely diseased.

In this book, we are concerned with these structures because some believe that they may (rarely) contract excessively (spasm), obstruct the ducts, and

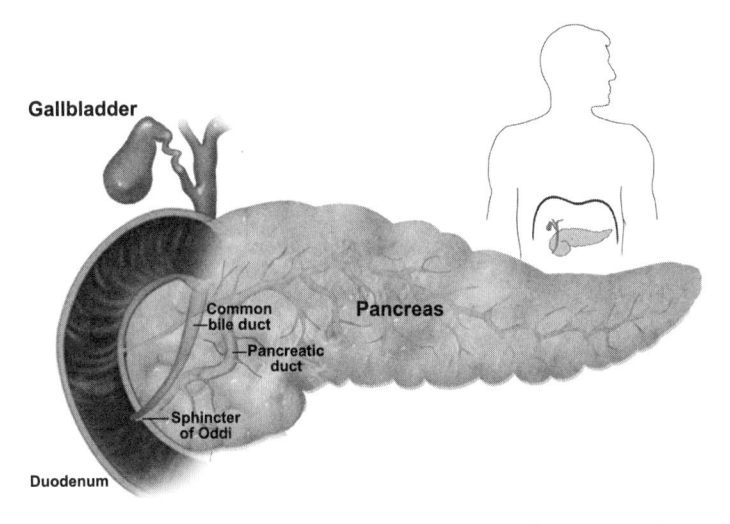

Figure 3-4. The pancreatic and biliary systems. The common bile duct and the pancreatic duct empty through the sphincter of Oddi into the duodenum. In a few people the pancreatic duct empties separately.

cause pain that resembles biliary or pancreatic disease. These painful syndromes are called the *functional gallbladder* and *sphincter of Oddi disorders*.

The Anorectum

The *rectum* is the terminal segment of the colon that stores feces in anticipation of their evacuation through the anus at a time convenient to its owner. The *anus* (sometimes mistakenly referred to as the rectum) includes the valve at the nether end of the gut that is the final determinant of continence. It includes an involuntary inner band of smooth muscle known as the *internal anal sphincter*. This sphincter responds to rectal filling by relaxation, which is a prelude to defecation. However, by willfully contracting skeletal anal-muscle fibers known as the *external anal sphincter,* one can arrest that process—at least until the concert ends.

But this is not the end of the continence story. As shown in figure 3-5, a muscular sling known as the *puborectalis* pulls the rectum forward at the point where it joins the anal canal to create an anorectal angle. This acts as a further check to impromptu evacuation, and it must relax to permit orderly defecation. Disordered function of this muscular sling is believed to be at least partly responsible for some functional anorectal disorders, including *proctalgia fugax* and *dyssynergic defecation*.

Neurogastroenterology

According to *Rome III*, "Neurogastroenterology encompasses the investigative sciences dealing with functions, malfunctions, and malformations of

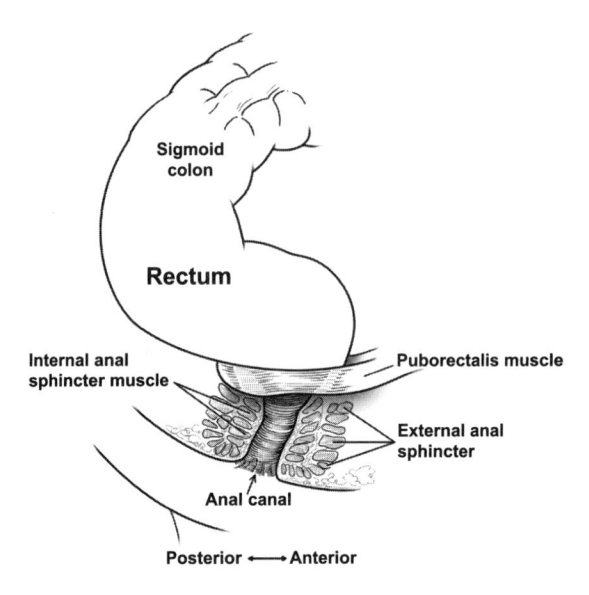

Figure 3-5. The anorectum. Note that the puborectalis muscle is contracted to create the anorectal angle. As the muscle relaxes, the anorectum straightens. The internal anal sphincter must then relax if defecation is to occur. The voluntary muscle of the external anal sphincter is the last barrier to defecation.

the brain and spinal cord and the sympathetic, parasympathetic, and enteric divisions of the autonomic enervation of the musculature, glands, and blood [vessels] of the gastrointestinal tract." Applied neurogastroenterology, the clinical application of this science, involves clinical testing of the gut's function. This comprises the use of tests that measure gut activity, and the development of drugs designed to ameliorate gut dysfunction. This is the basic science of the FGIDs. In the *Rome III* book, chapters 2 through 4 address the science in great detail. Here we present a brief overview to permit understanding of how intestinal function is controlled, what dysfunctions might occur in the FGIDs, and how interventions may be designed to correct them.

The Enteric Nervous System

The enteric nervous system (ENS), a division of the autonomic nervous system, is situated within the walls of the digestive tract and provides independent integrative neural control of digestive functions. The *sympathetic* and *parasympathetic* are the other divisions. The ENS, sometimes called the "gut brain," has many of the brain's attributes. It is capable of initiating and coordinating certain programmed, but subconscious, gut functions and it shares many of the brain's chemical mediators such as acetylcholine and serotonin.

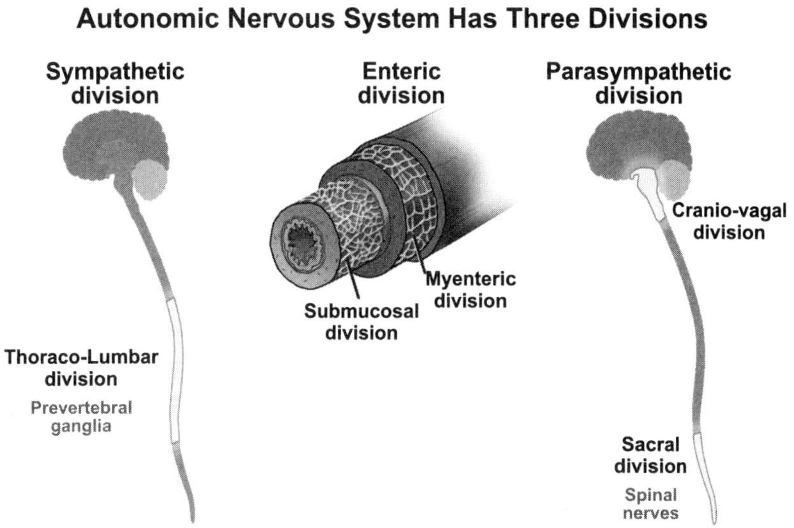

Autonomic Nervous System Has Three Divisions

Sympathetic division

Thoraco-Lumbar division
Prevertebral ganglia

Enteric division

Submucosal division
Myenteric division

Parasympathetic division

Cranio-vagal division

Sacral division
Spinal nerves

Figure 3-6. The digestive tract is innervated by the autonomic nervous system and by sensory nerves projecting to the spinal cord and brain stem. The sympathetic, enteric, and parasympathetic divisions of the autonomic nervous system constitute the autonomic innervation. Sympathetic and parasympathetic pathways transmit signals between the central nervous system and the gut. These are the extrinsic components of innervation. Neurons of the enteric division form the local control networks within the gut wall; they are the intrinsic components of innervation. The figure illustrates the enteric nervous system lying as nerve plexes within the layers of the gut wall. These plexes are sometimes known as the "gut brain." Comprehensive autonomic innervation of the digestive tract consists of interconnections between the brain, the spinal cord, and the enteric nervous system. (From Wood JD, 2003)

The ENS is indicated in figures 3-6 and 3-7. There are two nerve complexes, the *myenteric plexus*, lying between the inner circular and the outer longitudinal muscles of the gastrointestinal tract, and the *mucosal plexus*, lying within the inner muscle layer, beneath the gut's inner lining, the *mucosa*. Nerve ganglia contain the cell bodies of nerve cells whose long, slender processes connect with one another and with the muscle and endocrine cells that they sense and control. These nerve fibers or *axons* coordinate muscle contractions throughout the length of the gastrointestinal tract to produce complex movements called peristalsis. *Secretomotor nerves* connect to the mucosa where they provide neuroendocrine control of absorption and secretion.

In addition to motor or effector nerves that supervise the gut's functioning, *sensory nerve fibers* transmit impulses from specialized sensors such as those

Table 3-1. Some Neurotransmitters Found in the Enteric Nervous System and Their Functions

Motility	Visceral Sensation	Secretion
Serotonin (5-HT)	Serotonin (5-HT)	Serotonin (5-HT)
Acetylcholine	Tachykinin	Acetylcholine
Nitric oxide	Calcitonin gene-related peptide	Vasoactive intestinal polypeptide (VIP)
Substance P	Neurokinin A	
Vasoactive intestinal polypeptide (VIP)	Enkephalins	
Cholecystokinin (CCK)	Corticotrophin-releasing factor (CRF)	
Corticotrophin-releasing factor (CRF)		

Adapted from the *Rome III* slide set

that detect pressure or stretch within the gut wall. These connect to motor fibers that participate in local reflexes and to the central nervous system (CNS) via the spinal cord. The latter connections account for our gut feelings.

Like computer programs, subconscious ENS programs direct electrical nerve transmissions to release or activate various chemical neurotransmitters and hormones that cause target cells to react. These may signal smooth-muscle contractions or release hormones and digestive enzymes. Transmissions in the opposite direction activate reflexes and permit us to sense discomfort, pain, and other gut symptoms. Some of the many neurotransmitters that function in the ENS are listed in table 3-1. Current pharmacological research is focused on these chemicals. Drugs that augment or block these neurotransmitters could have profound therapeutic (or harmful) effects upon gut function. While some of these interventions may improve certain symptoms, none are curative, and as yet no precise ENS derangement has been identified to explain any of the FGIDs.

The Brain-Gut Axis

The ENS is capable of independent function, such as the "programmed" relaxation of the LES to let swallowed material pass, or intestinal peristalsis to move material towards the anus. We are normally unaware of such activity. However, the brain is not a disinterested bystander. There are comprehensive connections between the ENS and the CNS via the spinal cord. Centers in the base of the brain transmit both excitatory and inhibitory motor impulses to

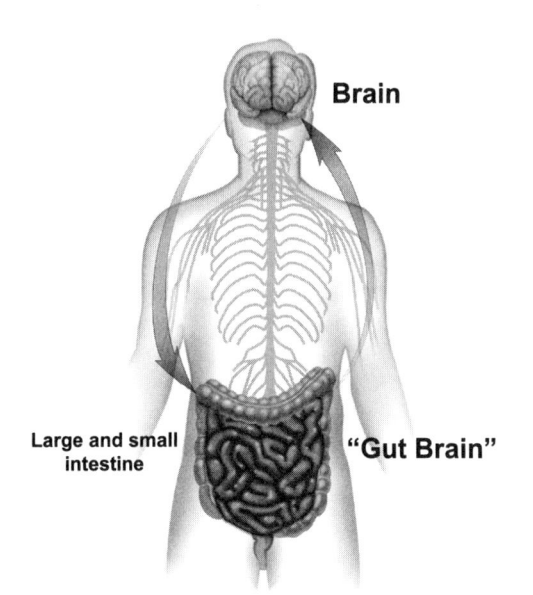

Figure 3-7. The brain-gut axis refers to the communication between the central and enteric nervous systems.

Brain

Large and small intestine

"Gut Brain"

the gut via these connections, and they in turn are governed by impulses from the brain's higher centers, such as the cerebral cortex.

In this way, sensation, thought, and emotion can have subtle influences on gut function. The smell and taste of food stimulates the stomach to secrete acid and enzymes. Extreme emotion can alter gut function as well. Who has not experienced "butterflies," diarrhea, nausea, or maybe vomiting during a stressful experience? It is through such visceral sensation that central influences may unconsciously contribute to functional gut disorders. A current hypothesis suggests that in the FGIDs the gut is "hypersensitive." This visceral hypersensitivity may be a normal reaction to an abnormal stimulus (hyperalgesia) or an abnormal reaction to a normal stimulus (*allodynia*).

While digestion and absorption of nutrients normally proceed silently, abnormal muscle contractions, or muscle stretch receptors stimulated by distension of the intestines, may send impulses up the spinal cord to centers in the brain where they are recognized as discomfort or pain. Thus, the brain-gut nerve traffic is two-way, and significant events at one end of the brain-gut axis are unlikely to be ignored by the other. Noxious sensations generated in the intestines are quickly recognized by the brain, where they may profoundly affect an individual's emotions and thinking. Alternatively, emotional and mental turmoil in the brain may profoundly affect gut function. We do not know the cause of FGID symptoms, but any explanation must take into account this dynamic interaction between brain and gut. Meanwhile, any treatment plan must address disturbances in both organs.

30   Understanding the Irritable Gut

Peristalsis

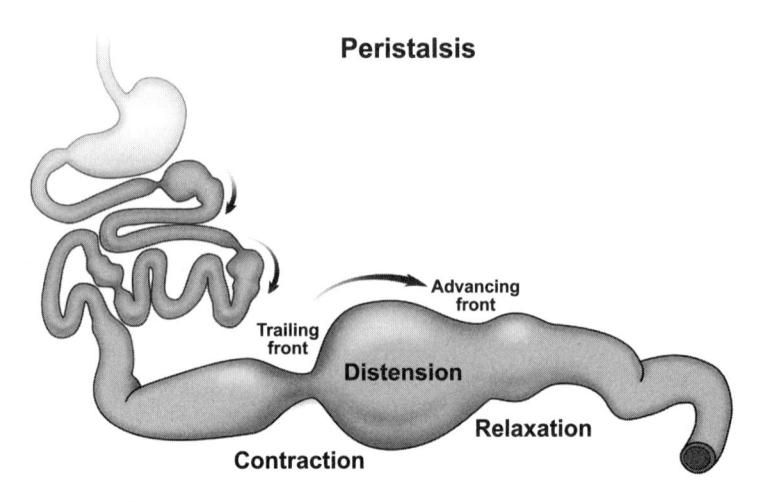

Figure 3-8. Peristalsis. A progressive wave of gut muscle contraction is preceded by relaxation, thus moving intestinal contents along.

Gut Motor Function

The gastrointestinal tract has two smooth muscle coats, an inner circular layer that contracts to squeeze the intestinal contents, and an outer, longitudinal layer that shortens and lengthens a gut segment as it contracts and relaxes. Under the neural and chemical influences discussed above, these gut muscle layers act in a highly organized manner to move ingested material along in a manner that supports the digestion and absorption of nutrients. The fundamental movement is peristalsis (see figure 3-8). The esophagus, stomach, small intestine, and colon, each in its own way employs peristalsis to empty itself.

A peristaltic wave comprises an advancing circular muscular contraction and longitudinal foreshortening. The circular muscle relaxes ahead of a bolus of food and contracts behind it, propelling it away from the mouth. Esophageal transit is a rapid and normally one-way response to a swallow. The filled stomach stimulates its distal part, the *gastric antrum*, to send repetitive peristaltic waves against the contracted pylorus to grind and mix the food. Gradually the mixed food is squirted into the small intestine in a state that is now fit for digestion. Small intestinal peristalsis is intermittent, with pendulous back and forth mixing over hours to facilitate digestion of food and absorption of its nutrients. Left-sided colon and sigmoid peristalsis periodically sweeps contents to the rectum in a state fit for defecation.

There is a series of muscular valves that act as gates along the gastrointestinal tract. They include the upper and lower esophageal sphincters, the pylorus, the ileocecal valve, and the internal and external anal sphincters. Uniquely, the first and last of these sphincters contain skeletal muscle that is under voluntary control. The remaining involuntary sphincters, under neuroendocrine and local reflex control, relax to permit the passage of food and digested material and, in the case of the LES, contract to prevent reflux of gastric acidic contents into the esophagus.

Conclusion

The gastrointestinal tract is a complex, smooth muscle organ under the control of the enteric nervous system or gut brain. The ENS is connected to the brain by ascending sensory pathways. Descending stimulant and inhibitory pathways influence gut function. At both ends of the brain-gut axis, common chemical mediators such as serotonin and acetylcholine transmit neural messages. The FGIDs are classified according to the segment of the gastrointestinal tract where their symptoms are believed to originate: the esophagus, the gastroduodenum, the intestines, the pancreatic and biliary ducts, and the anorectum. Each has a unique set of physiologic functions that can become disordered. When the cause and precise nature of such a dysfunction is not understood, the disorder is deemed "functional."

Sources

Camilleri M, Bueno L, De Ponti F, Fioramonte J, Lydiard RB, Tack J. Pharmacological and pharmacokinetic aspects of functional gastrointestinal disorders. In: Drossman DA, Corazziari E, Delvaux M, Spiller RC, Talley NJ, Thompson WG, Whitehead WE, eds. *Rome III: The Functional Gastrointestinal Disorders.* McLean, VA: Degnon Associates, Inc.; 2006:161-229.

Kellow JE, Azpiroz F, Delvaux M, Gebhart GF, Mertz H, Quigley EMM, Smout AJPM. Principles of applied neurogastroenterology: physiology/motility-sensation. In: Drossman DA, Corazziari E, Delvaux M, Spiller RC, Talley NJ, Thompson WG, Whitehead WE, eds. *Rome III: The Functional Gastrointestinal Disorders.* McLean, VA: Degnon Associates, Inc.; 2007:89-159.

Wood JD. Neurogastroenterology and digestive motility. In: Rhoades RA, Tanner GA, eds. *Medical Physiology.* 2nd ed. Baltimore: Lippincott Williams & Wilkins; 2003:449-480.

Wood JD, Grundy D, Al-Chaer ED, Aziz Q, Collins SM, Ke M, Taché Y. Fundamentals of neurogastroenterology: basic science. In: Drossman DA, Corazziari E, Delvaux M, Spiller RC, Talley NJ, Thompson WG, Whitehead WE, eds. *Rome III: The Functional Gastrointestinal Disorders.* McLean, VA: Degnon Associates, Inc.; 2006:31-87.

4 What Causes the Functional Gastrointestinal Disorders?

Introduction

Inherent in any definition of the functional gastrointestinal disorders (FGIDs) is that their causes and mechanisms are unknown. When a disorder is assigned a cause, it is no longer called "functional." For example, a disease called *achalasia,* where food accumulates in the esophagus, might once have been called "functional." Indeed its original name was cardiospasm, since early x-rays suggested that the cause was obstruction due to spasm in the lower esophageal sphincter (LES). However, we now know that achalasia is due to both a failure of the lower esophageal sphincter to relax and a failure of lower esophageal peristalsis to clear the organ, caused by damaged enteric nerves in the wall of the esophagus. With the structural cause so precisely known, the LES can be forcibly opened by a dilating instrument and the swallowing difficulties can be ameliorated. For these reasons, achalasia is not considered an FGID. Although we may suspect that spasm or failure of relaxation may cause some of the FGIDs, we can neither prove it nor logically direct remedial therapy.

Theoretical Causes of the FGIDs

Nevertheless, the FGIDs do not lack theories. There are too many to catalogue them all here, but some are especially important. A few of these hypotheses are vigorously supported by their protagonists, and some may be true in some cases. The theories may be grouped as physiological, psychosocial, nature versus nurture, environmental, bacteriological, and "visceral hypersensitivity." Most of the available data relates to irritable bowel syndrome (IBS), but said data are often extrapolated to the other disorders. These putative causes will be discussed where appropriate in part 2, but some general observations are appropriate here.

Physiological Theories

It is obvious that the gastrointestinal tract behaves abnormally in the majority of people with FGIDs. With such symptoms as diarrhea, constipation, and vomiting, it cannot be otherwise. Thus abnormal gut motility has long been recognized to underlie these disorders. For half a century, investigators have struggled to measure the gut's complex movements in largely vain attempts to distinguish abnormal from normal. Three facts stand in the way of a physiological explanation. First, except for the esophagus and anorectum, current technology is difficult to apply in the gut, and gut motility analyses so far have failed to explain FGID symptoms. For centuries, spasm of the colon was believed to cause the pain of IBS, but no test can consistently confirm this.

Second, any observed motility disorder in an FGID would not tell us *why* it occurred. Evidence is accumulating that any abnormality must involve the complex neuromuscular and neuronsensory apparatus of the enteric nervous system and its interactions and shared chemistry with the brain and spinal cord. Moreover, the whole system may be disturbed by other factors such as stress, mood, and diet. Finally, while the motility characteristics in some FGIDs such as IBS and constipation are often observed to be abnormal, others such as functional heartburn and functional abdominal pain exhibit no evidence of dysmotility at all. Even putative upper esophageal sphincter and puborectalis abnormalities are far from proven to cause globus and proctalgia fugax.

Research in gastrointestinal motility has done much to explain some abnormalities at the gut ends, such as achalasia in the esophagus, and Hirschsprung's disease, where the rectum's lack of nerves causes severe constipation. Motility studies will undoubtedly help identify specific abnormalities in some disorders that we currently consider functional. However, by themselves motility measurements do not help us understand most FGIDs.

In chapter 3, we described the many chemical neurotransmitters in the enteric nervous system (ENS). These permit sensory and motor signals to and from the gut. Not only are their activities controlled and reported via connections to the brain, but many of these gut peptides are also found in the brain itself. For more than half a century, the research focus was on acetylcholine, since this neurotransmitter substance is plentiful in the gut and its pharmacological activation or antagonism has profound effects on gut behavior. Anticholinergic drugs that block the action of acetylcholine can improve diarrhea and, because they can paralyze the gut, they were thought to be useful in reducing pain due to gut spasm. However, their efficacy (and the relevance of gut spasm itself) remains unproven, and because their side effects are considerable, few experts now recommend them.

In the last two decades, attention has been focused on serotonin and its several receptors in the gut, as well as in the brain. Could a fundamental defect in serotonin metabolism explain FGIDs, and could drug intervention put it right? Researchers are encouraged by the great success of centrally acting, serotonin-affecting drugs in the treatment of depression and other psychological disorders. If they work in the brain, why would they not do so in the gut? Certain of these drugs slow or accelerate gut transit and thus may offer antidiarrhea or laxative capability. Moreover, there is evidence that antidepressants themselves alleviate some FGID patients' symptoms. However, as yet there is no evidence that derangements of serotonin or any other gut chemical are solely responsible for any FGID, and the above-mentioned treatments are palliative rather than curative.

There are many neurotransmitters in the ENS and its brain connections (see table 3-1). These provide great scope for pharmaceutical research and are the most likely targets of new drugs to treat the enigmatic FGIDs. The utility of such interventions does not necessarily depend upon whether an ENS or neurotransmitter malfunction causes a disorder. Rather, by inhibiting or enhancing normal function they may correct a troublesome symptom such as diarrhea, vomiting, or visceral hyperalgesia.

Psychosocial Theories

Much research relates to the psychological disturbances that are found in patients with FGIDs. However, it is important to keep the data in perspective. Most of the research has been done by specialists or psychologists seeing referred patients who are not responding well to the care of their primary care physicians (see figure 2-5). As discussed in chapter 2, it is not clear that the resulting published data are germane to most primary care patients or to those who in surveys are found to have an FGID, yet never see doctors. Indeed, the psychological states of individuals with FGIDs who have not consulted physicians are similar to those individuals without these disorders. While psychosocial factors do not define the disorders and are not required for their diagnosis, they can greatly influence the patient's experience and behavior—and ultimately the outcome of treatment. Many patients suffer disorders such as depression, anxiety, and panic. The FGIDs, at least in specialty care, are often accompanied by significant life stresses, and by a history of physical or sexual abuse. Since nonpatients in the community with functional symptoms are psychologically similar to people without such symptoms, one cannot safely ascribe the FGIDs to psychosocial disturbances. Nevertheless, the degree of psychosocial disturbance intensifies the impact of the symptoms and the degree of daily impairment.

Thus, remembering the biopsychosocial model, psychosocial factors can greatly determine how a patient is affected by his symptoms and how he behaves. Whether these factors exacerbate the symptoms themselves through the brain-gut interconnections, or by increasing a person's awareness of the symptoms and exaggerating their importance (hypervigilance), they are vitally important to confront if the management plan is to be successful. It should not be forgotten that FGID symptoms can be chronic and very troublesome, in which case they may themselves induce psychosocial stress. Thus, a person's gut symptoms and psychosocial state may interact and conspire to make him feel worse than if the two factors were simply added together. Patients may be caught in a vicious cycle where years of distress from a chronic functional disorder lead to anxiety and distress, precipitating flare-ups, amplifying the intensity of the experience, and further aggravating the physiological disturbance. Psychological treatment may help the patient cope with this vicious cycle.

Finally, it has been observed that physical and emotional stress can precede the onset of FGID symptoms—or at least the reporting of them to a doctor. In such a case, addressing the factors that caused the stress prior to the doctor visit is as important as the management of the physical symptoms. Acute or chronic stress may not cause the symptoms, but may greatly affect patients' suffering and ability to cope.

Nurture versus Nature Theories

The children of adults with IBS are likely to have more gut symptoms than others, exhibit more anxiety and depression, and visit doctors more frequently. Symptoms and health care-seeking may be learned from parents, or the family's diet, stresses, and lifestyle may contribute to the development of FGIDs. Moreover, if a child is rewarded for illness through avoidance of school, extra television, and other favors, he may be inclined as an adult to expect analogous treatment.

However, twin studies suggest that there is also a genetic or inherited basis for FGID symptoms and illness behavior. There are numerous neurochemical and inflammatory pathways that might express a genetic predisposition to gut symptoms. The relative importance of inheritance and early childhood experience in the development of functional disorders is unknown. Existing evidence suggests that both are important.

Environmental Theories

When a person has a chronic gut disorder and symptoms occur, it is natural to attribute them to something she has eaten. However, the interpretation of an individual's food-related symptoms is difficult. The stomach, intestines, and colon all begin to contract after meals so as to empty themselves and prepare for the receipt of the next meal (the *gastrocolonic response*). In an already irritated or sensitive gut, these gut contractions, or a person's perception of them, may be exaggerated after a meal, even if it is perfectly bland. Often it is the quantity of food consumed that causes problems, rather than its nature. In either case, the meal's content erroneously may be blamed for a symptom, and be avoided inappropriately when it may be better to eat less or eat more slowly. Nutrition may be threatened if many foods are withdrawn in this fashion.

Among organic diseases, more specific dietary disorders include celiac disease, where one must avoid grain products that contain gluten to prevent intestinal damage, weight loss, severe nutritional deficiencies, and diarrhea. People who lack the enzyme lactase in the cells that line the jejunum will have limited tolerance to the milk sugar known as lactose, and will suffer diarrhea and bloating if they drink too much milk. Consumption of contaminated food may induce an enteric infection, but cannot explain the repeated attacks of an irritable bowel. In some people, ingestion of fatty foods predicts a sensation of bloating and fullness after meals. Conversely, those with peptic ulcers often feel their dyspepsia when the stomach is empty and its acid content is not buffered by food. Overeating, junk foods, and eating too rapidly are all capable of upsetting the digestive system, or aggravating an already irritable gut. These possibilities require attention whether or not an FGID is present.

Much is made of the notion that food allergy is responsible for FGID symptoms. Sensitivity to such items as shellfish, certain nuts, and strawberries is dramatic and verifiable. However, in only a very few patients does a food allergy trigger the characteristically chronic and recurrent symptoms of an FGID. Nevertheless, some people with FGIDs may appear to be sensitive to something in their diet. Some diet reactions may accompany an FGID without necessarily being the cause. While improvement can be expected if these reactions are attended to, complete cure is unlikely. In most cases no specific dietary cause of an FGID is identified, and dietary restrictions offer little relief over the long term. Ingested material is the most credible putative environmental cause of an FGID, but others are blamed. These include respiratory allergens, bad air in buildings, and extremes of weather. Such theories are unproven and largely untested.

Lifestyle characteristics such as lack of exercise, uncontrolled work stress, irregular eating and defecation habits, and lack of sleep may not cause IBS symptoms, but can aggravate them. Mundane examples include a constipated patient's "insufficient time" for defecation, or a dyspeptic person's power lunch.

Inflammation and Bacteriological Theories

Doctors have always regarded the colon bacterial flora with suspicion. Although they are useful to us metabolically and defend us immunologically, some of our bacterial tenants may become pathogens and induce disease. The interface between colon bacteria and the intestine's inner wall is an immunological war zone, since even normally friendly colon organisms can wreak havoc if they enter the gut's tissues or the blood vessels that richly supply it with nutrients. Scientists question how secure the barrier is to colonic bacteria, and wonder whether some FGIDs could be chronic infectious diseases or persisting out-of-control immune reactions to resident, but not-so-friendly bacteria.

In some cases of IBS, investigators report increased inflammation in the lining or mucosa of the intestine and in the neural plexes that lie beneath. This is suggested by an increase in activated inflammatory cells and the chemical mediators of inflammation. These may perturb gastrointestinal reflexes and activate the visceral sensory system. The apparent development of IBS symptoms and some residual inflammation after enteric bacterial infections suggests that inflammation-related IBS may be induced by bacterial enteritis. Up to a quarter of IBS patients relate the onset of their symptoms to an infection, especially those due to *Shigella* or *Campylobacter* bacteria. However, we cannot be certain that all such cases were truly without symptoms prior to their infection. An enteric infection raises a person's awareness of any gut disturbance. Such an infection likely increases one's susceptibility to gut symptoms both physiologically and psychologically.

In the belief that the colon flora may be hostile, many advocate treatment of gut symptoms with so-called probiotics. These are normally harmless organisms that can be cultured and packaged as capsules in preparation for their ingestion as treatment for such disorders. "Bad" bacteria may cause microscopic inflammation that could sensitize the enteric sensory nerves. By introducing "good" bacteria, one can presumably crowd out the putative bad ones and relieve the symptoms.

Another theory is that the normally almost sterile small intestine becomes overgrown with bacteria that are not normally resident there. Some investigators report such overgrowth in IBS patients more often than in others. However, few believe these data explain the symptoms for most FGID patients. The use of antibiotics to treat such patients is fraught with undesirable and sometimes dangerous side effects. More research is necessary to substantiate this hypothesis.

Visceral Hypersensitivity

Many FGIDs such as IBS, esophageal chest pain, and functional dyspepsia are characterized or dominated by pain. Research has failed to discover any physiologic phenomenon to explain the pain. This leads many researchers to believe that individuals with such complaints have amplified visceral sensation. As we have seen, the viscera (in this case the intestinal organs) are richly supplied with sensory nerve endings that have extensive interconnections with the enteric nervous system and hence the spinal cord and brain.

Experimentally, when a balloon is inflated within the rectum, some but not all IBS patients perceive pain at lower inflation pressures than normal people. Some scientists suggest that this *visceral hyperalgesia* explains why patients with the painful FGIDs seem to report greater than expected pain with noxious stimuli. Perhaps they have increased sensitivity to even normal function, a phenomenon called *allodynia*. Amplification of gut sensations could occur in the enteric nervous system, in the areas of the body surface where the sensations are felt, in the nerves in the gut, in connections with the central nervous system, or in the brain itself via the spinal cord. Further, an increased appreciation of an enteric stimulus could result from failure of the normal pain-inhibiting impulses from the central nervous system. Perhaps stress or emotional disturbances impair the brain's ability to inhibit noxious gut sensations. Research shows that repeated noxious stimuli increase the pain, and suggests that maybe the hypersensitivity can be learned or acquired from repeated insults. Chronic abdominal pain may be the end result of such a process. Similar phenomena might also amplify nonpainful symptoms such as bloating or heartburn.

Visceral hypersensitivity might result from a variety of physiological and psychological insults including infections (postinfectious IBS), abnormal gut flora, ingested toxins, stress, and early childhood experiences. In fact, visceral hypersensitivity can serve as an all-embracing theory for any of the factors discussed in the previous sections or shown in figure 1-2.

The notion that visceral hypersensitivity explains the FGIDs is a theory, not a fact. However, it is a very useful one. It provides hypotheses for experimental research. It encompasses most other credible scientific theories, and it provides an understandable framework for explaining the disorders to patients. Moreover, it lends credibility to the diet and lifestyle adjustments necessary to remove factors that may aggravate a hypersensitive gut. These include stress, poor diet, and inadequate time for defecation. Whether this currently attractive theory prevails will depend upon the outcome of future research. Thomas Almy summed up the riddle many years ago; "Is the IBS [or any FGID] a normal reaction to abnormal gut physiology, or an abnormal reaction to normal gut physiology?" Or is it both?

Conclusion

The causes and mechanisms of the FGIDs are poorly understood, although many theories are vigorously promoted. Physiological, psychological, inherited, environmental, infectious, and other influences are regularly observed by doctors, but none offers a comprehensive explanation. Perhaps several of these interact in an individual. Visceral hypersensitivity offers a credible and overarching theoretical framework for the symptoms, and is the basis of much contemporary study. It embraces most other theories, and is a useful concept to stimulate research and explain the conditions to patients. Furthermore, it legitimizes the condition by providing a plausible explanation for the symptoms that goes beyond the dismissal that they are "in my head." Progress in our understanding is slow, but that does not mean we are ignorant. As the *Rome III* book attests, we know much about normal gut function and how to recognize each disorder, the nature and behavior of the FGIDs, their aggravating factors, and how to manage them. Over many years, the stimuli for the acquisition of this knowledge have been theories and hypotheses. By testing these, new observations are made, knowledge expands, and new ideas come to mind. Theories and hypotheses are important, even if they eventually prove to be untrue.

Sources

Almy TP. The irritable bowel syndrome: back to square one? *Dig Dis Sci.* 1980;25:401-403.

Drossman DA. Treatment for bacterial overgrowth in the irritable bowel syndrome. *Ann Intern Med.* 2006;145(8):626-628.

Drossman DA. The functional gastrointestinal disorders and the *Rome III* process. In: Drossman DA, Corazziari E, Delvaux M, Spiller RC, Talley NJ, Thompson WG, Whitehead WE, eds. *Rome III: The Functional Gastrointestinal Disorders.* McLean, VA: Degnon Associates, Inc.; 2006:1-30.

Drossman DA, Corazziari E, Delvaux M, Spiller RC, Talley NJ, Thompson WG, Whitehead WE, eds. *Rome III: The Functional Gastrointestinal Disorders.* McLean, VA: Degnon Associates, Inc.; 2006.

Gwee KA, Graham JC, McKendrick MW, Collins SM, Marshall JS, Walters SJ, Read NW. Psychometric scores and persistence of irritable bowel after infectious diarrhoea. *Lancet.* 1996;347:150-153.

Levy RL, Jones KR, Whitehead WE, Feld SI, Talley NE, Corey LA. Irritable bowel syndrome in twins: Heredity and social learning both contribute to etiology. *Gastroenterology.* 2001;121:799-804.

Spiller RC. Estimating the importance of infection in IBS. *Am J Gastroenterol* 2003; 98:238-241.

Thompson WG, Heaton KW. *Fast Facts: Irritable Bowel Syndrome*, 2nd ed. Oxford: Health Press; 2003.

Whitehead WE, Crowell MD, Heller BR, Robinson JC, Schuster MM, Horn S. Modelling and reinforcement of the sick role during childhood predicts adult illness behaviour. *Psychosom Med.* 1994;56:541-550.

PART 2 The Functional Gastrointestinal Disorders: Nature and Diagnosis

Introduction

The functional gastrointestinal disorders (FGIDs) are classified according their presumed anatomical origins: esophagus, gastroduodenum, bowel, pancreaticobiliary tree, and anorectum (table 1-1). This classification directs diagnostic and therapeutic attention to the affected part of the gut. Part 2 describes the individual FGIDs, beginning in chapter 5 by describing how they are diagnosed.

The *irritable bowel syndrome* (IBS) is the most studied FGID, and accordingly has validated diagnostic criteria. Moreover, some data exist to enable evidence-based IBS therapy. Because many people consider IBS to be the prototypical FGID, it is discussed first in chapter 6. *Functional constipation* (chapter 7) troubles many people and can be stubborn. It must be differentiated from organic disorders, some of which are themselves uncommon and poorly understood. *Functional diarrhea* deserves its own chapter (chapter 8), not because it is very common, but rather because it may diagnosed only after meticulous testing for known causes of chronic diarrhea.

Functional dyspepsia, described in chapter 9, is difficult to define and in the past was referred to as nonulcer dyspepsia. Although the upper abdominal pain and discomfort in ulcer and functional dyspepsia may be similar, experts are reluctant to describe one as simply the absence of the other. Successive Rome working teams have made the diagnosis more inclusive and have altered the classification, subtypes, and criteria of functional dyspepsia, demonstrating that the Rome process is a work in progress.

Chapter 10 describes the functional esophageal disorders—among the few FGIDs that are best diagnosed by exclusion. If the symptoms of heartburn, chest pain, dysphagia, or globus fail to respond to powerful gastric acid-suppressing drugs, acid-sensitive gastroesophageal diagnoses are excluded and the illness is likely to be functional. The functional anorectal disorders (chapter 11) are particularly troublesome to patients. Physiological tests are helpful, but not yet sufficient to reliably define these disorders or predict their treatment. The remaining disorders, discussed in chapter 12, are also important, but less common and less studied. Management options for the FGIDs appear in Part 3.

5 How Are the Functional Gastrointestinal Disorders Diagnosed?

Introduction

Diagnosis is the art and science of identifying the diseases that cause a person's physical abnormalities and symptoms. It is a vital part of the medical process because only by identifying the disease can doctor and patient bring to bear what has been learned about it and institute rational or evidence-based treatment. In organic disorders diagnosis can be confirmed by testing, such as radiographic imaging or blood analyses. Diagnosis is no less important in the functional gastrointestinal disorders (FGIDs), where there is no confirmatory test. Seeking and making a diagnosis are essential in FGID management. However, the lack of physical identifiers may seem to make diagnosis uncertain. This chapter will address the special considerations that accompany a functional diagnosis, the importance of making such a diagnosis confidently, and the means by which the diagnosis can be made.

Diagnostic Considerations in the Functional Gastrointestinal Disorders

In chapter 1, we used the example of dyspepsia to illustrate the difference between functional and organic diseases. Peptic ulcer dyspepsia can be explained by discovering the peptic ulcer through an endoscope. When an ulcer or other disorder cannot be found, we say that the dyspepsia is "functional." That does not mean the dyspepsia has no cause, but rather that science has yet to elucidate one. Even known organic diseases may present in obscure ways, and occasionally a person is said to have a functional disorder until the cause is finally identified. Because FGIDs are very common, it should not surprise us that organic and functional disorders may coexist in an individual. Crohn's disease, for example, is characterized by severe gut symptoms relating to bleeding, obstruction, or abscess. However, functional gut symptoms sometimes intervene, even when the Crohn's is inactive. The treatment of these two chronic disorders is very different, so a doctor must accurately interpret the patient's symptoms.

Because some organic diseases are deemed disabling and life-threatening, many doctors feel compelled to do too much testing to "rule them out." While it is certainly important to identify mortal disorders, the *Rome* authors believe that usually the FGIDs can be identified by a careful history, a physical examination, and a minimum of tests. Of course, people at special risk of organic disease must be carefully scrutinized, but excessive testing can be counterproductive. Medical tests are expensive, not without risk, and if excessively pursued can generate anxiety and insecurity about the correct diagnosis.

The Importance of a Diagnosis

Diagnosis is art *and* science. It is a skill that receives much, yet not enough, attention in medical school. Since this is not a clinical text, suffice it to say that the vital and intellectual task of diagnosis cannot be delegated, hurried, or computerized. However, it is germane to point out the contribution of the Rome process to the diagnoses of the FGIDs. The *Rome* criteria for the individual disorders appear in appendix A, and can be used to help doctors diagnose their patients' functional complaints.

At first glance, a precise FGID diagnosis seems unnecessary, since no pathology is revealed and no precise treatment is available. By exclusion, there is nothing seriously wrong. Surely, the important thing is that no disease has been demonstrated! This approach is wrong for several reasons. First, as the *Rome III* book emphasizes, a diagnosis is possible on the basis of an interview, an examination, and a minimum of tests. An exclusive approach implies that all other diseases have been ruled out by conducting too many tests that may expose the patient to unnecessary risks and expense. Even when another disease is present, it is important to recognize accompanying functional symptoms so that they will not be treated inappropriately. In the above example, if functional gut symptoms are attributed to Crohn's disease, potentially dangerous drugs such as steroids may be wrongly prescribed.

Second, an FGID diagnosis focuses the investigation. Dyspepsia in most cases will indicate a stomach and duodenum examination, while functional bowel disorders should focus attention on the intestines. There are many possible organic causes for gut symptoms. A *Rome III* diagnosis, by localizing the dysfunction, can shorten the list of possible diseases and limit the tests.

Third, scientific research concerning the tests and treatments of the FGIDs requires precise criteria to classify the patients who are entered into studies. Subsequently, only by applying these same criteria to their patients can doctors know to whom the resulting scientific data apply.

However, the most important reason for providing patients with an FGID diagnosis is to properly inform and reassure them. While we might be relieved to hear that our symptoms do not mean debilitating disease or death, we are dissatisfied if we are simply told there is nothing wrong. After all, the symptoms are real and their dismissal will not abolish them. Diagnosis is an essential part of treatment. By telling an FGID patient what is known of his disorder, a physician provides a construct for him to understand his symptoms. The diagnosis implies that the complaints have been encountered before and that the product of that experience may help provide some relief. It is unlikely that any modern doctor has said that a patient's FGID is "all in the head," but lack of diagnosis, a pat on the back, and insistence that nothing is wrong can transmit that demeaning message all the same. Many people with FGIDs fear cancer, yet are reluctant to use the "C" word. If the doctor fails to recognize this, patients may leave the clinic fearful and forget whatever else they are told. By providing meaning for a patient's symptoms, doctors offer a context or rationale and hold out the possibility that, now that we know the nature of the disorder, management can begin. In busy office practices doctors may fail to make a diagnosis and explain it. Patients should insist upon it.

How Diagnoses Are Made

Diagnosis and treatment are intertwined. They both commence with the medical interview and consolidate as doctor and patient become comfortable with each other and the facts surrounding the illness emerge. Although the processes of diagnosis and treatment should not be separated in practice, it is useful here to consider the elements of diagnosis alone. In the following chapters, we will discuss the individual FGIDs, and their diagnosis will be part of that discussion. In Part 3, diagnosis and treatment will come together as we describe the management of the FGIDs. Throughout the *Rome III* book, the authors stress the importance of a successful therapeutic relationship between doctor and patient.

The Medical History

For all diseases, but especially for the FGIDs, an accurate and thorough history is the key to correct diagnosis. By using the data compiled by generations of physicians and by recruiting her experience and skill, a physician mentally tests the diagnostic possibilities as the consultation progresses. Of course, she will seek out the chief complaint and the history of the symptoms related to that complaint, but meanwhile she will consciously and subconsciously gather all sorts of relevant information that contributes to the formulation of a diagnosis. Diagnosis is both an art of disclosure and a science of probabilities. It is impossible to be right all the time. Even during the interview, a doctor must change the diagnosis if certain facts intrude to invalidate the original conclusion. Accumulating information about the patient's gender, age, ethnic background, social position, occupation, and family status may shift the possible diagnoses from one set of diseases to another. Meanwhile, the physician's eyes are alert to signs of physical disease, and of anxiety, depression, anger, or other emotion that may influence the complaint.

It is often speculated that computers might gather such data through programmed questionnaires. However, no computer can extract and weigh medical evidence as well as the human mind. Only by direct interview can a doctor assess the relative severity of the symptoms and the patient's response to them, while observing the mood and concern with which he conveys this information. It seems an irony that some people suggest employing lesser-trained nurse-practitioners for this most demanding of medical tasks, while the doctor does something more useful!

Physical Examination

After the medical interview, a doctor usually has a good sense of the diagnosis, or has selected the two or three most likely possibilities. The physician may focus the physical examination according to the patient's complaint, but he is usually not surprised by the findings. In the case of the FGIDs, there are no physical findings. A lump in the abdomen, or an enlarged liver, or a heart murmur cannot be explained by a functional disorder. Therefore, such findings should prompt further inquiry and testing. Conversely, the discovery of physical disease through attention to alarm symptoms (table 5-1) and physical findings does not negate the coexistence of functional symptoms that may require treatment alongside the organic disease.

The value of a physical examination cannot be underestimated. Not only may it clarify the history and help determine whether a structural disorder is

Table 5-1. Alarm Symptoms

Blood in the stool or black stools
Vomiting blood
Low blood count (anemia)
Fever (>38 degrees Celsius, 99 degrees Fahrenheit)
>5 kilograms (10 pounds) weight loss
Recent major change in frequency or consistency of bowel movements
Parent or sibling with cancer of esophagus, stomach or colon,
Ulcerative colitis, Crohn's disease, or celiac disease
Recent, persistent hoarseness
Recent, persistent, or worsening throat pain
Chest pain related to exertion or present with heart disease
Recent onset of difficulty swallowing

Adapted from *Rome III: The Functional Gastrointestinal Disorders*, pp. 934-936.

Table 5-2. Psychological Alarm Symptoms

Tense or "wound up" (anxiety)
Downhearted and low (depression)
So low that one feels like hurting or killing oneself (suicide ideas)
Great bodily pain (severity)
Symptoms interfere with normal activities including work (impairment)
"It is terrible and I feel it will never get better" (impaired coping)
Emotionally, physically, or sexually victimized (abuse)

Adapted from *Rome III: The Functional Gastrointestinal Disorders,* pp. 955-959.

present, but it may also serve as treatment in itself. For a patient who is fearfully enduring a painful symptom, it is a comfort to have the affected part carefully examined by an expert. "At last, someone is taking my symptoms seriously!" Previously in agony, a patient may visibly relax with confident examination of the affected part. Surgeons call it "the laying on of hands."

Investigation

When the interview and physical examination are complete, the doctor will have decided whether the disorder is likely to be organic or functional and, considering such things as age, gender, family history, and alarm symptoms (table 5-1), will select the appropriate tests. At this point, some explanation is due the patient. If the doctor suspects IBS or another FGID, she should indicate this to the patient, if necessary recommend one or two tests to be sure no other disease is present, and explain that the tests will likely be negative. It is not enough to simply order tests and provide a diagnosis. The doctor must also explain what the test results and diagnosis mean.

Many people with FGIDs need no testing. In a young person with typical symptoms, no physical findings or alarm symptoms, no other disease or drug treatments, and no suspicion or family history of another illness, a comprehensive interview and examination alone permit a confident diagnosis. Older people are more liable to mortal diseases such as cancer, so those over forty-five with bowel symptoms should have a colon examination. Dyspeptic symptoms may merit an endoscopy to rule out a curable peptic ulcer.

Patients should ask why the tests are being done. Moreover, they should understand that a negative test is usually good news, and does not merely deepen the mystery. A normal test result makes a mortal or physically debilitating disease less likely and builds confidence in an FGID diagnosis. Once accomplished, a diagnosis enables doctor and patient to work together to ameliorate the symptoms.

Psychological Comorbidity

Many patients with FGIDs who consult physicians have psychological or social problems that need attention if their biopsychosocial needs are to be properly addressed. It is therefore important to recognize associated anxiety, depression, or other psychological disorder. Table 5-2 indicates psychological alarm symptoms that may help with this recognition. As with other aspects of the medical history, recognition requires patience and careful listening.

The Follow-up Visit

Doctors often arrange a follow-up appointment to assess the patient's response to advice or treatment. Such a visit also provides an opportunity to gather any further evidence that might change the diagnosis and to assess how well the patient has understood and reacted to the doctor's explanation of the symptoms. A family doctor is particularly well positioned to judge the external factors that bear on a patient's illness and to arrange appropriate follow-up observation.

Conclusion

The diagnosis of an FGID should not be arrived at only after an exhaustive battery of tests designed to exclude every possible organic disease. Rather, it should be formulated as the physician conducts a medical interview and physical examination. Patients with alarm symptoms and some who are elderly may require one or two tests and follow-up visits to confirm the absence of an organic disease. An early, confident diagnosis permits the doctor to allay a patient's worst fears and begin the education essential to successful self-management. Diagnosis *is* treatment!

Sources

Almy TP. The irritable bowel syndrome: back to square one? *Dig Dis Sci*. 1980;25:401-403.

Brody H. The lie that heals: the ethics of giving placebos. *Ann Int Med*. 1982;97:112-118.

Talley NJ. *Conquering Irritable Bowel Syndrome*. Hamilton, ON: B.C.Decker, 2005.

Thompson WG, Heaton KW. *Fast Facts: Irritable Bowel Syndrome*, 2nd ed. Oxford: Health Press; 2003.

6 Irritable Bowel Syndrome

Irritable bowel syndrome is a functional bowel disorder in which abdominal pain or discomfort is associated with defecation or a change in bowel habit, and with features of disordered defecation.
—Rome III: The Functional Gastrointestinal Disorders

Introduction

The irritable bowel syndrome (IBS) is the most important of the functional gastrointestinal disorders (FGIDs). It is not the most common—functional heartburn, bloating, and constipation may be more common—but IBS is the most studied and appears to generate the greatest share of health care costs. According to many surveys employing different populations and diagnostic criteria, it affects from 7% to 20% of adults in a year and the lifetime prevalence is likely to be much higher. However, these figures can mislead. Most people who admit to having IBS in surveys do not seek medical attention and apparently do not consider themselves ill. Nevertheless, those who do seek help constitute a significant part of medical practice. Not only are they responsible for about 2% of adult primary care visits and perhaps half of a gastroenterologist's practice, but also they are subject to much expensive testing, unjustified hospitalization, and mistaken abdominal and gynecological surgery.

Direct medical costs incurred by IBS patients in the United States are estimated to be $1.9 billion. Indirect costs through work loss and nonmedical treatments are almost $20 billion. Patients with IBS have an impaired quality of life and frequent comorbid psychological and somatic complaints. These facts make a positive, efficient diagnostic approach imperative. The lack of a known cause and the plethora of purported treatments, none of which are curative, invite a conservative management approach, which will be discussed in part 3.

Diagnosis
How is IBS Recognized?

The sine qua non of IBS is abdominal pain. Because there are many other causes, the pain often presents a diagnostic challenge. Hence the frequency of gallbladder, appendix, and gynecological operations that appear to be prompted by IBS rather than a diseased organ. Other abdominal diseases such as Crohn's disease may occur in patients who also have IBS, or who were mistakenly thought to have IBS. Some doctors speak of "pelvic pain" as if it were specific to the reproductive organs. However such pain, felt in the lower abdomen, may be due to IBS. Therefore, the term "pelvic pain" provides no help to diagnosis and may direct one away from the recognition of intestinal symptoms. The nature of the abdominal pain is the key to diagnosis. The definition cited at the beginning of this chapter states that the abdominal pain or discomfort is associated with defecation or a change in the bowel habit and with disordered defecation. What this means is that the pain is often relieved when the patient has a bowel movement, or that the frequency and consistency of the stool changes when the pain occurs. Thus, with IBS pain, the stools become looser and more frequent or firmer and less frequent—features that have led to the concept of *diarrhea-dominant IBS* and *constipation-dominant IBS*. These IBS features are captured in the *Rome III* diagnostic criteria (table 6-1).

The *Rome III* criteria also provides a threshold of frequency (at least three days/month in the last three months), and stipulates that the symptoms be present for at least three months. A requirement of six months since onset is added to exclude transient symptoms or acute intestinal infections. Certainly, IBS must start sometime and can be present for a shorter period. However, it is normally encountered as a chronic disease and should not be confused with acute infections.

Alarm symptoms germane to IBS are listed in table 6-2. These cannot be explained by the IBS and indicate a risk of significant pathology. If present, they require some investigation.

For a young person with IBS symptoms who has no alarm symptoms and a normal abdomen determined by physical examination, a diagnosis may be made with minimal or no investigations. If alarm symptoms exist, or if the patient is older and therefore liable to other diseases such as colon cancer, certain tests are indicated. However, typical IBS symptoms are not those of colon

Table 6-1. Diagnostic Criteria* for IBS

Recurrent abdominal pain or discomfort** at least three days/month in the last three months associated with *two or more* of the following:
1. Improvement with defecation
2. Onset associated with a change in frequency of stool
3. Onset associated with a change in form (appearance) of stool

* Criteria fulfilled for the last three months with symptom onset at least six months prior to diagnosis
**"Discomfort" means an uncomfortable sensation not described as pain.
Rome III: The Functional Gastrointestinal Disorders, p. 491

6. Irritable Bowel Syndrome   51

Table 6-2. Alarm Symptoms for IBS

Blood in the stool or black stools
Vomiting blood
Low blood count (anemia)
Fever (>38 degrees Celsius, 99 degrees Fahrenheit)
>5 kilograms (10 pounds) weight loss
Recent major change in frequency or consistency of bowel movements
Parent or sibling with colon cancer
Ulcerative colitis, Crohn's disease, or celiac disease

Adapted from *Rome III: The Functional Gastrointestinal Disorders*, pp. 934-936.

cancer. That disease is equally likely to be present in those with IBS and those without; often cancer has no symptoms at all until very late in the progress of the disease.

Stool Form

The most important indicator of diarrhea and constipation is the stool form, or consistency. Frequent passage of hard stool is pseudodiarrhea, not diarrhea, and infrequent loose stools in the absence of laxatives is not constipation. Figure 6-1 illustrates the *Bristol Stool Form Scale*. By identifying her stool's appearance on this scale, a patient enables her doctor to determine whether she

Type 1
  Separate hard lumps, like nuts, hard to pass
Type 2
  Sausage shaped, but lumpy
Type 3
  Like sausage, but with cracks on surface
Type 4
  Like sausage or snake, smooth and soft
Type 5
  Soft blobs with clear cut edges
Type 6
  Fluffy pieces with ragged edges, a mushy stool
Entirely liquid
Type 7
  Watery, no solid pieces

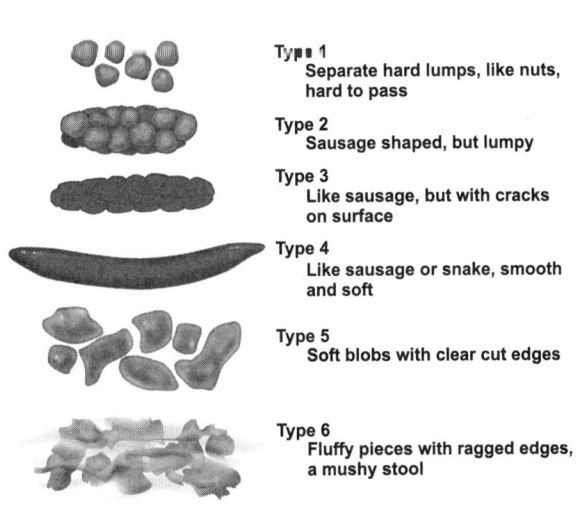

Figure 6-1. The Bristol Stool Form Scale. (Adapted from Heaton KW et al., 1991 for *Rome III: The Functional Gastrointestinal Disorders*)

Table 6-3. Subtyping IBS by Predominant Stool Pattern

To subtype patients according to bowel habit for research or clinical trials, the following subclassification may be used (see figure 6-1 and figure 6-2). The validity and stability of such subtypes over time is unknown.

1. IBS with constipation (IBS-C)—hard or lumpy stools[a] >25% *and* loose (mushy) or watery stools[b] <25% of bowel movements*
2. IBS with diarrhea (IBS-D)—loose (mushy) or watery stools[b] >25% *and* hard or lumpy stool[a] < 25% of bowel movements*
3. Mixed IBS (IBS-M)—hard or lumpy stools[a] >25% *and* loose (mushy) or watery stools[b] >25% of bowel movements*
4. Unsubtyped IBS—insufficient abnormality of stool consistency to meet criteria for IBS-C,D, or M*

---

* In the absence of antidiarrheal or laxative use
[a] Bristol Stool Form Scale 1-2 (Separate hard lumps like nuts [difficult to pass] or sausage-shaped but lumpy)
[b] Bristol Stool Form Scale 6-7 (Fluffy pieces with ragged edges, a mushy stool or watery, no solid pieces, entirely liquid)
(A fifth subtype [IBS-A] describes patients who switch subtypes from time to time.)
Adapted from *Rome III: The Functional Gastrointestinal Disorders*, p. 492.

---

has diarrhea or constipation (assuming the patient has not taken antidiarrhea medication or laxatives). Table 6-3 and figure 6-2 demonstrate how an IBS patient's bowel habit can be characterized by using this scale. This characterization helps to ensure that treatment will be appropriate.

IBS Subtypes

Because most therapeutic agents promoted for IBS have either an antidiarrhea or laxative activity, it has become common to subtype IBS into those with diarrhea (*diarrhea-dominant IBS*) or constipation (*constipation-dominant IBS*). However, the most predictable feature of the bowel habit in IBS patients is its unpredictability. Over time both diarrhea and constipation will manifest in many people with IBS; there may be periods of neither, or both. Therefore, the *Rome III* bowel committee thought it prudent to change the terminology to *IBS with diarrhea (IBS-D)* and *IBS with constipation (IBS-C)*. Two other categories, *mixed* and *unsubtyped IBS*, are important for research, but need not concern us here. While IBS itself is a stable diagnosis that seldom changes over time, the subtypes are less constant. An individual who changes between IBS-D and IBS-C is called an alternator (*IBS-A*). Drugs with antidiarrhea or laxative activity should be used according to the patient's bowel habit at the time of treatment. A recorded diagnosis of IBS-C could lead to inappropriate laxative treatment should the bowel habit change.

Rome III IBS Subtypes: Stool Form

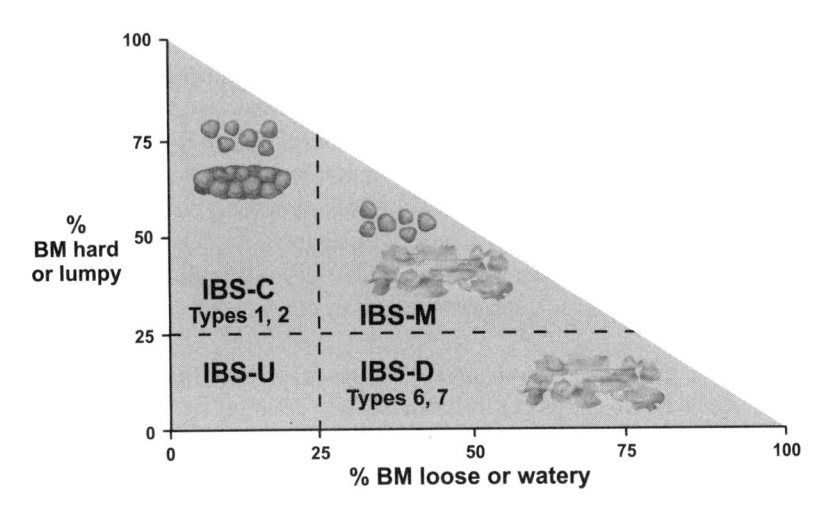

Figure 6-2. Two-dimensional display of the four possible IBS subtypes according to the current stool form. BM = bowel movement, IBS-C = IBS with constipation, IBS-D = IBS with diarrhea, IBS-M = mixed IBS, IBS-U = untyped IBS. Not shown is alternating IBS (IBS-A), where the subtype changes over time. The classification threshold is 25%. In the case of IBS-C, that means that more than 25% of bowel movements are types 1 or 2 according to the Bristol Stool Form Scale. In the case of IBS-M, more than 25% of bowel movements are types 1 or 2, *and* more than 25% are types 6 or 7. (Adapted from *Rome III: The Functional Gastrointestinal Diseases*, p. 493.)

Other Diagnoses to Consider

The alarm symptoms listed in table 6-2 cannot be explained by IBS; they demand further inquiry. Blood in the stool is a very important symptom. Bright red blood appearing through the anus that coats or streaks the stool usually is caused by an anal disease such as tear (anal fissure) or hemorrhoids. However, there are a number of serious diseases that also may cause colon bleeding. The most important is cancer of the colon or rectum. In North America and Europe, colon cancer becomes more common after the age of fifty, especially in people with siblings or parents with the disease. Often bleeding is the only symptom. The presence of IBS offers no protection against colon cancer, so bleeding in an elderly person with or without IBS mandates a colonoscopy to exclude a cancer or precancerous benign tumor (polyp). Abdominal pain due to cancer usually means bowel obstruction, which can be a surgical emergency, or invasion into other tissues that requires analysis through computed tomography (CT) or magnetic resonance imaging (MRI).

Also in the elderly, severe, often constant abdominal pain and fever may mean diverticulitis. Diverticular disease describes the occurrence of rows of berry-sized outpouchings in the colon called *diverticula*. These occur in at least 50% of Western adults by age seventy, and normally cause no symptoms. The presence of IBS symptoms with diverticular disease is coincidental, but both conditions are common in the elderly and therefore commonly occur together. Occasionally a diverticulum bursts and becomes infected, resulting in an acute, febrile illness with severe abdominal pain that requires antibiotics and occasionally surgery. Sometimes diverticulitis may be subacute and grumble along for a while with fever and pain—but it should never be confused with IBS. Unusually, one of the outpouchings may bleed, sometimes catastrophically so.

In the young, and less commonly in the old, rectal bleeding may be the first indication of ulcerative colitis or Crohn's disease. These inflammatory bowel diseases (IBD) are usually characterized by diarrhea, often accompanied by fever, weight loss, anemia, and a profound whole-body illness—features unlike those of IBS. Such symptoms mandate a colon examination and often investigation of the small bowel by ultrasound, barium contrast small-bowel enema, or CT. There are specific, effective, but sometimes potentially harmful treatments for these diseases, so it is essential that the symptoms not be confused with those of IBS. A physician's diagnostic skill is challenged to determine whether abdominal pain and diarrhea in a patient with IBD are due to the IBD itself or to coincidental IBS, lest the patient receive inappropriate drugs or surgery. As in the case of colon cancer, a family history of IBD increases the risk, and is therefore an alarm.

Lactose intolerance occurs in certain individuals of European descent, but is most common in non-Europeans. The disaccharide lactose is milk sugar, which consists of two primary sugars (monosaccharides), glucose and galactose. The latter are easily absorbed in the small intestine, but first they must be released from the lactose molecule by an intestinal enzyme called lactase. Insufficient intestinal lactase permits lactose to travel to the colon where the resident fecal bacteria feed upon it to produce gas (hydrogen) and short-chain fatty acids that cause diarrhea. The resulting gas, bloating, and diarrhea sometimes may be confused with IBS. A hydrogen breath test can help with the diagnosis, but substantial improvement on a milk-free diet is more convincing. One can make up the lost dietary calcium by ingesting yogurt, a milk product that contains no lactose.

Some gastroenterology clinics report that IBS symptoms may occur with celiac disease. This disease is common in the inhabitants of northern Europe and their descendents. It makes sense to test for celiac disease in Caucasian IBS patients where the disease is common, such as in Ireland and northern England, or where there is a deficiency of a nutrient such as iron or folic acid.

Celiac disease can be detected by a blood test for a specific antibody and confirmed by an intestinal biopsy taken with a gastroduodenoscope. The treatment of celiac disease is a rigid, expensive, and restricting diet that excludes the wheat protein gluten. Because the antibody test may be falsely positive, no one should embark on such a diet until the disease is confirmed by the typical microscopic features of celiac disease in an intestinal biopsy. Although there are anecdotal reports of improvement of IBS on a gluten-free diet, they are unconfirmed. Sometimes a short trial of therapy may be justified, but patients should not stay on such a diet indefinitely unless the symptoms greatly improve and repeatedly recur when gluten ingestion is resumed. Of course, IBS can occur with (not because of) celiac disease, as it can with any other condition.

Sometimes enteric infections causing diarrhea, gassiness, and abdominal cramps are chronic and may be confused with IBS. The parasite *Giardia lamblia* is an example. The presence of the parasite is difficult to diagnose, although an antibody test may help. Sometimes, *Giardia* is suspected in someone from an endemic area such as Russia, from a developing nation, or in someone who has camped near a contaminated lake. A physician may recommend a course of the antibiotic metronidazole regardless of the test result.

Investigation

Prior to the Rome attitude of a positive diagnosis, IBS was considered a "diagnosis of exclusion;" that is, it was an interpretation of abdominal symptoms arrived at only after many tests excluded every other abdominal condition. The *Rome* authors believe that approach is mistaken. The tests are costly, anxiety-producing, and sometimes harmful. Too often, when tests are repeatedly negative, the patient gets the feeling that his symptoms are not taken seriously, especially if no diagnosis is given.

The most important diagnostic test for IBS and its competing diagnoses is the clinical history. Only through a thorough analysis of symptoms using the *Rome* criteria and alarm symptoms can one recognize IBS and be alerted to the possibility of other disease. Routine blood tests are usually normal, but may reveal an unsuspected anemia, nutritional deficiency, or other abnormality that prompts further investigation. Older patients should have a colonoscopy to exclude colon cancer. If it were logistically possible, everyone in developed nations should have a colonoscopy around age fifty to detect this very preventable cancer. Benign colon polyps may be premalignant; because the cancer process takes many years, their removal can prevent a cancer. Other tests are indicated according to the IBS patient's circumstances, risk factors, and other relevant information gathered from the clinical history. In part 3 we will discuss treatment. However, diagnosis is the beginning of treatment, and patients should understand that in the context of IBS, negative tests are good news.

Comorbid Disease

IBS patients in specialist care or attending medical centers are likely to have coexisting somatic and psychological symptoms. The somatic symptoms are often functional disorders of other body systems such as headaches, fibromyalgia, chronic fatigue, and low back pain. They resemble the FGIDs in that they have no proven cause. These associations are less likely in primary care. This clustering of functional symptoms in referred IBS patients undoubtedly increases their sense of illness and reduces their quality of life. Perhaps several functional disturbances have a common cause, or they are found together in specialist care by coincidence. Perhaps they share a comorbid psychological condition. One study found that when a person with a cluster of functional symptoms seeks help, his diagnosis depends upon the first specialist he sees—a gastroenterologist sees IBS where a rheumatologist finds fibromyalgia. Whatever the explanation, patients require attention to *all* their symptoms, and some may be better cared for by a general physician than by several specialists.

Psychological disturbances are often intricately entwined with IBS, again especially among referred patients. It is uncertain whether such disorders cause IBS, provoke IBS, result from IBS, or simply coexist with and complicate IBS. The most common psychiatric diagnoses are depression, anxiety, and panic attacks. Whatever the mechanistic relationship of these conditions with IBS, the latter cannot be expected to improve unless the psychosocial issues are also managed. Table 5-2 lists psychosocial alarm symptoms that may help identify those patients with potentially serious psychological difficulties. Of course, these are just guides, but if present they require further inquiry—just as physical alarm symptoms do.

What Causes IBS?

Overview

In chapter 4, we reviewed the putative causes of the FGIDs, including IBS. Nevertheless, a few additional observations are appropriate here. We do not know the causes of IBS, nor what mechanisms generate the symptoms. Indeed, it is far from certain that it is primarily a bowel disorder. Many observers believe that the primary disturbance in IBS resides in the central nervous system, and that its transmissions through the enteric nervous system provoke the symptoms. Others believe the enteric nervous system itself is at fault, overreacting to the normal stimulation the gut receives as it goes about its daily work of digesting and absorbing food. Still others believe that some environmental factor is at work—an infection analogous to *Helicobacter pylori* that causes peptic ulcer, or a diet item like gluten that causes celiac disease. There are even some who view abnormal gut reactions in the absence of demonstrable disease as part of the human condition—a way in which our intestines respond to physical and psychosocial stresses. Any discussion of the possible causes of IBS must acknowledge that as yet there is insufficient knowledge to explain it, and that any current explanation is theoretical.

Finally, many believe that IBS may not be one disorder. There may be several causes. For example, prior to the discovery of lactose intolerance, many patients with that disorder might have been considered to have IBS. When it was discovered in the 1960s, enthusiasts predicted it would explain a quarter of IBS cases—in fact it explains very few. Some people with IBS and lactose intolerance have their IBS symptoms provoked by milk ingestion. There may be several other yet-to-be discovered ailments that together or separately explain some IBS flare-ups. The biopsychosocial model suggests that, in varying degree, many or all of the putative causes may together orchestrate IBS.

Intestinal Motility

Despite the half-century use of devices to measure the movements of the intestines, motility observations fail to explain how certain IBS symptoms such as abdominal discomfort or pain are generated. A further conundrum is the unpredictability of the gut's actions in IBS. As Cumming described it in 1849, "... the bowels are at one time constipated, at another lax in the same person. ... How the disease has two such different symptoms, I do not profess to explain...." Neither do I!

Of course, when someone with IBS is having diarrhea, we can surmise that the absorption of water is inhibited and increased peristalsis speeds evacuation of a watery stool. The opposite is likely the case with constipation. Nevertheless, studies of gut motility and secretion in IBS show inconsistent results and do not explain why the two extremes frequently occur in the same patient. In general, studies of patients who are diagnosed with IBS-D and IBS-C provide no definitive answer, and no data confirm that any abnormalities observed in these subtypes are stable over time.

The pain of IBS also is difficult to explain. For two centuries, undiagnosed gut pain was attributed to spasm of the colon or small intestine. However, careful study fails to identify a gut spasm that is unique to IBS, or to consistently demonstrate that pain occurs with spasm, but is absent without it.

A particular area of physiology research greatly influences thinking and carries us beyond motility as the basis for some of the gastrointestinal symptoms. That is the observation that IBS patients are more sensitive to inflation of a balloon within the rectum than are those without IBS. Reinforced by similar observations elsewhere in the gut, this phenomenon led to the now-popular theory of visceral hypersensitivity that is addressed below. These distension results may be a clue, but abnormal responses to distension are not reliably demonstrable in every IBS patient, and spontaneous distension has not been shown to occur simultaneously with IBS pain. It may be that changes in the tension within the gut wall stimulate local pain receptors.

Many believe that the secrets of IBS reside in the enteric nervous system

(ENS). Here numerous neurotransmitters and complex nerve ganglia supervise the normal management of gut activity. Perhaps abnormalities in how they communicate with the intestine and the brain can explain the chaotic gut behavior of IBS. To this end, many drugs have been developed to act on this system. However, it appears that such drugs, notably those directed to serotonin receptors, act in the ENS to promote increased or decreased peristalsis, so that their usefulness is limited to correcting the bowel dysfunction at the time of treatment. They do not address the IBS itself. Nevertheless, the ENS remains a fertile locus for useful new drug development.

Psychopathology
Another venerable theory is that the symptoms of IBS originate in the central nervous system—that is, that they have a psychological basis. This notion is encouraged by the depression, anxiety, panic, posttraumatic stress, sleep disturbance, and past physical and sexual abuse that are frequently observed in IBS patients who attend referral centers. However, relevant information from primary care and non-care-seeking IBS subjects in the community is scarce. Some community data suggest that there is either no such association or that the degree of psychological distress is modest. Moreover, not everyone with psychological distress has IBS.

The *Rome III* authors reject the psychosomatic theory that emotional conflicts cause FGIDs. Instead, the authors support the biopsychosocial model where management must take in all aspects of a person's illness, including the somatic complaints and the psychological state.

It may be that severe psychological stress triggers IBS symptoms via the central and enteric nervous systems. Another interpretation is that the psychopathology, not the IBS, prompts the patient's health care-seeking and eventual referral to a medical center—their gut symptoms merely direct them to a gastroenterology specialist. A further notion is that a person's psychological disturbance increases awareness of gut dysfunction that another individual might cope with or ignore. In any case, one cannot ignore the presence of psychosocial dysfunction in so many patients. Perhaps all of these possibilities alone or together help explain how psychosocial factors interact with IBS at various times in an individual. The ability to cope with IBS is unlikely to be improved until the psychological distress is alleviated.

Using complex technology such as positive emission tomography (PET) and functional magnetic resonance imaging (fMRI), the emotion and pain-modulating areas of the brains of IBS patients are seen to react uniquely to gut stimulation. This finding confirms that the brain participates in the reactions of the studied IBS patients, but is compatible with several interpretations, including visceral hypersensitivity.

Visceral Hypersensitivity

Chapter 4 discusses several theories of IBS causation. There, the notion of *visceral hypersensitivity* was introduced that could embrace most of these theories. That is, the IBS patient's brain is more aware of and alert to abnormal and even normal sensations emanating through changes in the gut and enteric nervous system than other people's brains are. What one person might ignore is experienced by a patient as discomfort or pain. Diarrhea and constipation might similarly be seen as overreactions to environmental stimuli. Such hypersensitivity might be induced by any putative psychological, infectious, inherited, or environmental cause.

The attractiveness of this all-embracing theory is that it provides a construct to help patients and doctors understand the condition. It is a rationale for a doctor to search for factors that may provoke a hypersensitive gut and try to manage them. Moreover, visceral sensitivity is a credible hypothesis to be tested by scientific research.

Conclusion

Although we do not know the precise causes of IBS, we do know much about its behavior in the community, its symptoms and quality-of-life disruption in individuals, the influences that may aggravate it, and how doctors may recognize it in the clinic. This information provides several opportunities that were not present two decades ago. Clinicians, patients, and researchers can now communicate IBS data using a common language. Subjects who are entered into clinical trials are identified by criteria that can also be used to identify similar patients in the clinic. A doctor can provide a diagnosis that not only focuses a patient's investigations, but also reassures him that the disorder is recognized, manageable, and not cancer. Diagnostic criteria have also helped us recognize that IBS is a public health problem that generates significant health costs, morbidity, and work loss. The accumulating data encourage enlightened approaches to IBS patients and removal of any stigma that the complaint is trivial, or "all in the head."

Sources

Almy TP. The irritable bowel syndrome: back to square one? *Dig Dis Sci.* 1980;25:401-403.

Cumming W. Electro-galvanism in a peculiar affliction of the mucous membrane of the bowels. *Lond Med Gazette.* 1849;NS9:969-973.

Heaton KW, Ghosh S, Braddon FEM. How bad are the symptoms and bowel dysfunction of patients with the irritable bowel syndrome? A prospective, controlled study with emphasis on stool form. *Gut.* 1991;32:73-79.

Longstreth GF, Thompson WG, Chey WD, Houghton LA, Mearin F, Spiller RC. The functional bowel disorders. In: Drossman DA, Corazziari E, Delvaux M, Spiller RC, Talley NJ, Thompson WG, Whitehead WE, eds. *Rome III: The Functional Gastrointestinal Disorders.* McLean, VA: Degnon Associates, Inc.; 2006:487-555.

7 Functional Constipation

Functional constipation is a functional bowel disorder that presents as persistently difficult, infrequent, or seemingly incomplete defecation, and that does not meet IBS criteria.
—*Rome III: The Functional Gastrointestinal Disorders*

Introduction
The prevalence of constipation depends upon the diagnostic criteria employed. The exclusion of IBS in the *Rome III* definition reduces prevalence figures considerably because many IBS patients are constipated. A survey of 731 women in south Wales used three definitions (figure 7-1): patient complaint; *Rome I* definition; and intestinal transit time as determined by the Bristol Stool Form Scale.* Although about 10% of the women had constipation by each of these definitions, only 2% were constipated by all three of them. Using the *Rome II* criteria and questionnaire, which excludes loose stools and the irritable bowel syndrome (IBS), a Canadian survey found constipation in 21% of adults, 26% in women and 15% in men. These figures seem too high, as it is unlikely that one-fifth of the population is pathologically constipated. It is uncertain how stable the diagnosis is—most people experience transient constipation. Nevertheless, constipation is a common clinical problem, and most patients have no recognizable cause. For that reason, they are said to have *functional constipation*. Studies agree that constipation increases with age and is more common in women.

Diagnosis
How is Functional Constipation Recognized?
The definition that introduces this chapter puts it nicely: constipation becomes a clinical problem when defecation is "persistently difficult, infrequent, or seemingly incomplete . . . " Nevertheless, the parameters of constipation are many, and the development of criteria that exactly express this description

---

* Transit time is related to the stool form. Hard stools (types 1 and 2) are associated with slow transit, while loose, watery stools (type 7) mean fast transit.

Constipation
By Three Definitions

Patient Perception — 63 people or 8.6%

Rome Criteria — 60 people or 8.2%

Slow Transit — 69 people or 9.4%

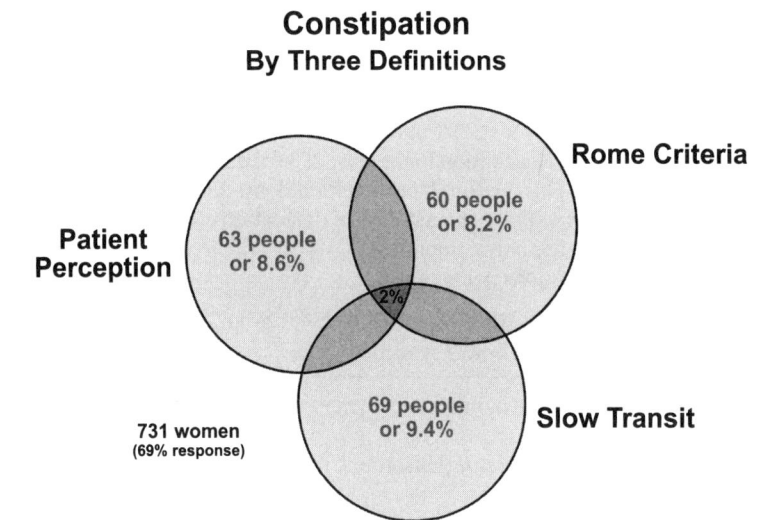

2%

731 women (69% response)

Figure 7-1. Prevalence of constipation in 731 women using three definitions (patient's perception, *Rome I* criteria, and gut transit as implied from the Bristol Stool Form Scale.) Each definition yields sixty to sixty-nine "constipated" patients—a prevalence of 8% to 10%. By at least one definition, 18% had constipation. Only 2% had constipation by all three definitions. (From Heaton KW et al, 1991.)

is complex. The *Rome III* criteria address constipation's many facets, requiring at least two of six possible characteristics (table 7-1). The first, straining, embraces the idea that defecation is difficult. The second describes the very important concept of stool form or consistency. The most reliable indicator of constipation is the continuous presence of stool types 1 and 2 on the Bristol Stool Form Scale (figure 6-1). Incomplete defecation is the basis of the third criterion. The fourth and fifth criteria in the list are designed to help identify patients who have anorectal dysfunction. A sensation of anorectal blockage and the use of manual maneuvers to free up stool suggest that if the usual treatments fail, the patient could be offered special anorectal motility studies. Infrequent defecation is a less reliable indicator of constipation. Hard and lumpy stools are associated with slow, not fast, intestinal transit. Therefore, even frequent passage of such stools is considered to be constipation. Nevertheless, "fewer than three defecations a week" remains as the sixth criterion.

Because the idea of persistence is important, the criteria must be present for at least six months. Transient constipation that is associated with hospitalization, travel, surgery, or acute emotional distress is not considered functional constipation, and is beyond the purview of this discussion. The exclusion of loose stools (unless the patient is using laxatives) also addresses the

Table 7-1. Diagnostic Criteria* for Functional Constipation

1. Must include *two or more* of the following:
   a. Straining during at least 25% of defecations
   b. Lumpy or hard stools in at least 25% of defecations
   c. Sensation of incomplete evacuation for at least 25% of defecations
   d. Sensation of anorectal obstruction/blockage for at least 25% of defecations
   e. Manual maneuvers to facilitate at least 25% of defecations (e.g. digital evacuation, support of the pelvic floor)
   f. Fewer than three defecations per week
2. Loose stools are rarely present without the use of laxatives.
3. Insufficient criteria for irritable bowel syndrome

*Criteria fulfilled for at least three months with symptom onset at least six months prior to diagnosis
Rome III: The Functional Gastrointestinal Disorders, p. 516

persistence issue. The exclusion of IBS is controversial and highlights the blurred demarcation between these two functional bowel disorders. IBS is characterized by abdominal pain that occurs with *altered* defecation. The distinguishing features of functional constipation are lack of pain and unchanging symptoms.

Other Diagnoses to Consider

As with all the functional gastrointestinal disorders (FGIDs), the medical history, fulfillment of *Rome III* criteria, and a negative physical examination provide the essential information to diagnose functional constipation. However, table 7-2 lists many causes of chronic constipation that must be considered in a full evaluation of a patient who presents with chronic constipation. Some of these causes are very rare, and quite often none of them apply. Nevertheless, they should be taken into account. There are contributing factors to be considered as well as three causative categories: constipating systemic diseases and their drug treatments, local colonic or anorectal disease, and functional defecation disorders.

The contributing factors include female gender—especially after hysterectomy, increasing age, general disability, depression, inactivity, many medications, and poor toilet habits. The inactivity, weakness, and dehydration that accompany a chronic illness such as depression, rheumatoid arthritis, or stroke may slow transit time and impair evacuation. Although specific measures such as laxatives must be employed, improvement depends more upon the successful management of the chronic disease and physiotherapy.

Hypothyroidism, depression, and several neurological conditions are systemic diseases that cause constipation through endocrine or neural derange-

Table 7-2. Causes of Constipation: Diagnosis and Specific Treatment

Pathology	Diagnosis	Specific Treatment
Drugs: opiates, psychotropics, anticonvulsants, calcium channel blockers, NSAIDs, calcium and iron supplements, anticholinergics, dopaminergics	History	Stop or switch to alternative medication
Endocrine disorder: diabetes mellitus, hypothyroidism	Clinical status, blood sugar, thyroid tests	Hormone replacement, surgery, etc.
Neurological diseases: diabetic neuropathy, Parkinson's disease, spinal cord lesion	History, neurological examination	Scheduled bowel training facilitated by suppositories or enemas
Slow transit due to neuropathy of colonic nerve plexus	Transit time, colon biopsy	Colectomy, if disease is confined to colon
Megacolon	X-ray	Colectomy if laxatives fail
Pelvic floor dyssynergia (anismus)	Proctoscopy, anorectal manometry, balloon expulsion, defecography, electromyography	Behavioral training, biofeedback training
Short-segment Hirschsprung's disease	Sphincter fails to relax with rectal distention, no ganglia on rectal biopsy	Internal anal sphincter myomectomy
Megarectum	X-ray	Enemas, laxatives
Internal rectal prolapse, solitary rectal ulcer	Proctoscopy, defecography	Fiber supplementation, surgery
Rectocele with stool retention	Proctoscopy, defecography	Nothing, transanal repair

Adapted from *Rome III: The Functional Gastrointestinal Disorders*, p. 520.

ment. The most common of the latter include Parkinson's disease, diabetic neuropathy, and spinal injury. In most cases, the cause is obvious, but others may require special tests. In the cases of hypothyroidism or depression, thyroid replacement or antidepressant therapy may be curative. Regrettably, many of the drugs used for neurological disease slow gut transit and further complicate the constipation. These include anti-Parkinson drugs, opiates (morphine, codeine), and tricyclic antidepressants. Table 7-2 lists some of many constipating medications. For examples, calcium channel-blocking drugs for hypertension, and nonsteroidal antiinflammatory drugs (NSAIDs) for arthritis cause constipation.

In general, colonic disease causes acute rather than chronic constipation. Examples are bowel obstruction due to cancerous or inflammatory obstruction of the intestines. The latter may include Crohn's disease in the young and severe diverticulitis in the elderly. Although these are usually subacute over a few weeks, they may provoke emergency surgery. Similarly, anorectal diseases such as an abscess or anal fissure are acutely painful, causing the patient to voluntarily withhold stool. Chronic constipation may occasionally result from a stricture of the anus due to chronic inflammation or anal fissure. Such abnormalities can be quickly recognized by anorectal examination, first with the doctor's examining finger, and later with a sigmoidosocope.

The remaining categories of constipating conditions are the functional defecation disorders that we will examine more closely in chapter 11. They include *inadequate defecatory propulsion* and *dyssynergic defecation* and are characterized by severe, intractable constipation. These uncommon disorders can be diagnosed through special tests in a medical center, under specialist supervision.

One's mental attitude to and physical attitude during defecation also must be considered. Many people find themselves too busy to visit the toilet, and deliberately rush the job. The result may be voluntary stool retention and poor evacuation. Moreover, although the Western toilet may be comfortable, it is less suited to the physiology of defecation than the squat, which remains the preferred attitude in most of the world. Bowel training to correct bowel habits is discussed in chapter 16.

Investigation

When it is established that a patient has persistently difficult, infrequent, or seemingly incomplete defecation, he should have routine blood analysis for anemia, inflammation (white blood count, C-reactive protein), and endocrine disturbances such as thyroid deficiency or high blood calcium. Most neurological conditions can be excluded by physical examination. In a young person without alarm symptoms, intestinal investigation is usually unnecessary beyond the anorectal examination discussed above. However, no constipated person over age fifty should fail to have a colon examination, preferably colonoscopy. Colon cancer is too common and too sinister to be missed, even if it is not the cause of the constipation. Table 7-2 suggests tests for the various disorders that might be suggested from the patient's history, or if the constipation is responding poorly to treatment.

One specific colon disorder, usually found in children, is a rare cause of chronic adult constipation. This is *Hirschsprung's disease*, which is characterized by a lack of nerve ganglia at the very lower end of the colon. Since surgery can be curative, the diagnosis should not be missed. Hirschsprung's can be recognized by a simple and sensitive measurement of internal anal sphincter relaxation in response to rectal balloon distension. If the test is positive and the ensuing rectal biopsy confirms the lack of ganglia, surgeons can revise the local anatomy to bypass the denervated segment.

Transit time

In severe, persistent constipation that is resistant to treatment, a dilemma presents itself. The diagnosis of the functional defecation disorders is difficult, expensive, and requires the services of a medical center with appropriately trained physicians and technologists. To a primary care physician contemplating referral of a persistently constipated patient to such a center, determination of colonic transit time offers a simple expedient that can be carried out at a local imaging (x-ray) facility. Several methods are described, one of which is the swallowing of twenty-five radiopaque markers followed by an abdominal x-ray five days later. If more than 20% of the markers remain in the colon, the transit time is deemed to be prolonged and may indicate further investigation. A similar test employs radioisotopes that emit less radiation than an x-ray, but that test requires a more sophisticated facility.

What Causes Functional Constipation?

Overview

Like IBS, functional constipation has no generally agreed-upon cause, and may turn out to have many causes. Indeed, many of the factors suggested in table 7-2 could be at work in a single person. In the individual case it is necessary to recognize them all if treatment is to be successful. Physiological, dietary, and psychological considerations are briefly discussed here.

Intestinal Motility

In most constipated patients, the colon transit time (a crude measure at best) is within the normal range, yet the hard stools, difficult defecation, and some experimental data suggest that it must be at the slow end of the normal range. As discussed above, two uncommon functional defecation disorders constitute extreme cases of functional constipation. *Inadequate defecatory propulsion* has a demonstrably slow colonic transit, sometimes accompanied by abnormal colon muscle or autonomic nerve function. Rarely, there are specific neurological or muscle disorders. In *dyssynergic defecation*, there is evidence of pelvic floor and anal dysfunction, meaning that there is resistance to the defecation process that leads to straining and a sense of difficult evacuation. Dyssynergic defecation, further discussed in chapter 11, is suggested by the fourth and fifth *Rome III* diagnostic criteria for functional constipation (table 7-1). These two uncommon types of extreme constipation may coexist.

Dietary Considerations

Dietary fiber has long been known to be an important component of normal defecation. Wheat products, especially wheat bran, have been known since the 1930s to increase stool weight and improve constipation. East African missionary doctors observed in the 1970s that constipation was rare among their patients who normally ingested a very high-fiber diet. Dietary fiber is the traditional first line of treatment for constipation. Besides increasing stool weight and bulk, fiber's bacterial digestion releases laxative short-chain fatty acids and gas that expands the stool. Despite these favorable observations, increased dietary fiber fails to reliably decrease transit time in severely constipated patients.

However, there is evidence that larger and softer stools do facilitate defecation. Using fabricated plastic feces, experimenters demonstrate that the smaller the stool, the more effort that must be expended to expel it. This may explain the slower passage of hard pellety stools (Bristol type 1). Such data underpin the use of fiber as the basic treatment of constipation. Indeed, fiber is cheap, easy to take, and often curative, so further measures are only required for those who fail to respond to it.

Although adequate hydration is recommended and seems to help some patients, there is no evidence that constipated patients are dehydrated. Nevertheless, because Bristol type 1 stools are dry, one should ensure adequate fluid intake. Similarly, physical exercise is deemed useful by doctors and the public alike. Although science has failed to confirm exercise's value, the extremes are instructive—inactivity due to illness is constipating, and long-distance runners are liable to diarrhea during a race.

Psychological Features

As in the case of IBS, constipated adult patients who are referred to medical centers may have associated psychological disorders. Whether these are cause, consequence, or coincidence is moot. Pathologically related or not, these associations are important to recognize if the doctor is to treat the constipated patient effectively.

Some children learn to voluntarily retain stool (*encopresis*), perhaps in response to imagined parental disapproval or some perceived secondary gain. Some data suggest that voluntary retention or faulty toilet training can lead to adult constipation or dyssynergic defecation. Experimentally, suppression reduces stool weight, stool frequency, and the urge to defecate, as well as prolonging colon transit.

Conclusion

There are many causes of and contributors to chronic constipation, but usually no single cause is discovered. The diagnosis is arrived at from the patient's clinical history using the *Rome III* criteria and the Bristol Stool Form Scale, along with a physical and anorectal examination. A diagnosis of functional constipation relies upon persistently difficult, infrequent, or seemingly incomplete defecation that does not meet IBS criteria, yet the common neural, endocrine, and pharmacological causes are excluded or corrected. In most young constipated people, little investigation is required beyond a few blood tests. Older patients require a colonoscopy to exclude colon cancer, even if there is no evidence of obstruction. A diagnosis of functional constipation embraces the functional defecation disorders to be discussed in chapter 11. Although there is no known cause of functional constipation, many possible contributing demographic, pharmacological, dietary, and disease factors must be investigated.

Sources

Heaton KW, Ghosh S, Braddon FEM. How bad are the symptoms and bowel dysfunction of patients with the irritable bowel syndrome? A prospective, controlled study with emphasis on stool form. *Gut.* 1991;32:73-79.

Longstreth GF, Thompson WG, Chey WD, Houghton LA, Mearin F, Spiller RC. Functional bowel disorders. *Gastroenterology.* 2006;130(5):1480-1491.

Wald A, Bharucha AE, Enck P, Rao AS. Functional anorectal disorders. In: Drossman DA, Corazziari E, Delvaux M, Spiller RC, Talley NJ, Thompson WG, Whitehead WE, eds. *Rome III: The Functional Gastrointestinal Disorders.* McLean, VA: Degnon Associates, Inc.; 2006:639-685.

8 Functional Diarrhea

Functional diarrhea is a continuous or recurrent syndrome characterized by the passage of loose (mushy) or watery stools without abdominal pain or discomfort.
—*Rome III: The Functional Gastrointestinal Disorders*

Introduction

The predominant feature of functional diarrhea is persistent, painless, loose, watery stools. The prevalence was determined to be 1.6% in a 1993 United States householders' study using the *Rome I* criteria, and 8.5% in a Canadian survey that used the *Rome II* criteria (table 2-1). In the clinic, however, true functional diarrhea is uncommon. It warrants a full chapter because, unlike many other functional gastrointestinal disorders (FGIDs), it must be identified from among several "organic" disorders that sometimes may be discovered only after repeat investigation. Unlike irritable bowel syndrome (IBS), it is a "diagnosis of exclusion"—chronic diarrhea demands investigation and follow-up.

Diagnosis

How Is Functional Diarrhea Recognized?

According to the *Rome III* criterion (table 8-1), the demarcation between IBS with diarrhea (IBS-D) and functional diarrhea is clear, because in IBS there must be defecation-related pain and functional diarrhea must be painless. In addition, functional diarrhea is persistent, affecting more than 75% of stools.

Most people, when asked what they mean by diarrhea, respond that their stools are loose or watery. This accords with the expert view that stool form or consistency is the critical identifying feature. The requirement that loose (mushy) or watery stools must present more than three-quarters of the time captures the persistence of diarrhea that characterizes functional diarrhea (table 8-1); these stool characteristics are a factor in all three *Rome* iterations. Unlike IBS-D, persistent diarrhea should prompt a careful and repeated search for the known causes of chronic diarrhea.

The absence of pain in functional diarrhea further differentiates it from

Table 8-1. Diagnostic Criterion* for Functional Diarrhea

Loose (mushy) or watery stools without pain occurring in at least 75% of stools

* Criterion fulfilled for the last three months with symptom onset at least six months prior to diagnosis
Rome III: The Functional Gastrointestinal Disorders, p. 524.

Table 8-2. Some Other Causes of Chronic Diarrhea

Diet	Chronic pancreatic insufficiency
Drugs	Crohn's disease
Lactose intolerance	Microscopic colitis
Bile acid malabsorption	Small-bowel bacterial overgrowth
Celiac disease	Villous adenoma
Giardiasis	Laxative abuse

Adapted from *Rome III: The Functional Gastrointestinal Disorders*, p. 525.

IBS. (Rarely, persistent diarrhea can occur with the features of IBS including pain, a circumstance or coincidence not accounted for in the criteria.) Nevertheless, any patient with loose, watery diarrhea occurring in more than three-quarters of defecations requires investigation whether pain is present or not. As with other functional bowel disorders, the Bristol Stool Form Scale can help patients and doctors identify the characteristic diarrhea stools (types 6 and 7 in figure 6-1). Sometimes, the frequent passage of hard, pellet-like stools may be mistaken for diarrhea (*pseudodiarrhea*)—a mistake the stool form scale helps avert. Alarm symptoms that are particularly important in patients with diarrhea include significant weight loss, blood and/or pus in the stool, fever, and a family history of inflammatory bowel disease (IBD).

Other Diagnoses to Consider

A shortened list of the many possible causes of chronic diarrhea is presented in table 8-2. A doctor will want to be sure they are absent before diagnosing functional diarrhea.

A careful diet history is especially important, beause many foods loosen the stools if taken in excess. Fructose, a sugar, is found in fruits, preservatives, soft drinks, and chocolate. Sorbitol is a sugar-free sweetener found in diet chewing gum, vanilla ice cream, and some medications. Caffeine is found in coffee, tea, and cola drinks. Each causes diarrhea if taken in excess. So too will excessive ingestion of alcohol, which impairs the absorption of sodium and water in the small intestine. If the offending agent is withdrawn from the diet, the diarrhea should disappear. Similarly, many drugs cause diarrhea, no-

Table 8-3. Some Drugs That Can Cause Chronic Diarrhea

Laxatives	Antibiotics
5-HT$_4$ agonists (tegaserod)	Alcohol
Antacids containing magnesium hydroxide	Caffeine
Herbal teas containing senna	Sorbitol
Misoprostol	

Adapted from Thompson WG and Heaton KW.

tably laxatives (table 8-3). Lactose intolerance may explain the diarrhea that occurs mainly in non-Caucasians who drink sufficient milk.

Bile salts, excreted from the liver into the duodenum, normally are reabsorbed into the blood from the ileum (figures 3-3 and 3-4). However, if the ileum fails to absorb them, the bile salts reach the colon, where they have a laxative effect. Thus a diseased ileum, or one surgically removed for Crohn's disease, fails to recapture the bile salts, thus causing *bile salt diarrhea*. Rarely, an apparently normal ileum may inexplicably fail to reabsorb bile salts. In such cases, ingestion of the bile salt-binding resin cholestyramine can dramatically decrease the diarrhea.

Diarrhea is the principle complaint of about half of patients with untreated celiac disease. With or without diarrhea, celiac patients often present with nutritional deficiencies because of malabsorption of iron, folic acid, calcium, or magnesium. Weight loss is common. Wholly treatable with a gluten-free diet, this diagnosis should not be missed. A positive blood test for antitissue transglutaminase (tTG-IgA) is very suggestive of celiac disease. The diagnosis must be confirmed by a duodenal biopsy obtained through an endoscope. Because its interpretation becomes unreliable after the diet is established, the biopsy should be done before committing a person to a costly and difficult-to-comply-with gluten-free diet.

The pancreas produces enzymes that are secreted into the duodenum where they digest fat and other nutrients. If these enzymes are deficient, they result in fat maldigestion and malabsorption that cause a type of diarrhea called *steatorrhea* (excess maldigested or malabsorbed fat in the stool). Replacing the enzymes in sufficient doses can improve diarrhea and digestion. Pancreatic insufficiency and celiac disease both cause steatorrhea.

Giardiasis is a parasitic infection that can cause chronic diarrhea. Stool examination for cysts is unreliable, so when there is suspicion, as after a trip to an area where the water supply is suspect, doctors may try a course of an antibiotic to kill any parasites that may be present.

Inflammatory bowel disease [IBD (Crohn's disease and ulcerative colitis)] is a common cause of diarrhea, but is usually recognized through alarm symptoms, a colonoscopic appearance of ulcerative colitis, or, in a patient with

Crohn's disease, the finding of a mass of swollen, inflamed small intestine. However, early in the disease alarm symptoms may not be evident and the lower colon may be uninvolved, especially in Crohn's disease. Therefore, in a developed country IBD must always be considered in a young person with chronic diarrhea. There are several possible reasons for the diarrhea: weeping of fluid from the inflamed intestine, failure to absorb bile salts as described above, bacterial overgrowth, and intestinal malabsorption due to extensive small-bowel disease. Improvement of the diarrhea depends upon successful management of the underlying IBD.

An uncommon variant of IBD known as microscopic colitis causes chronic diarrhea. As the name implies, it can be diagnosed only by microscopic examination of a colon biopsy taken through a sigmoidoscope or colonoscope. Treatment is imperfect, but sometimes patients improve on drugs that are normally used for IBD.

Bacteria may occasionally prosper in the normally sterile upper small intestine, especially in the elderly, or in those with a duodenal diverticulum or surgically induced intestinal cul de sac. Through impaired bile-salt metabolism and other mechanisms, the bacteria may cause chronic diarrhea and malabsorption of nutrients such as vitamin B_{12} and fat. Intermittent courses of an antibiotic may be necessary to suppress the bacteria. Chronic diarrhea due to small-bowel overgrowth is uncommon and difficult to prove, so good judgment is necessary to avoid unwarranted therapy and the adverse effects of antibiotics.

A *villous adenoma* is a usually benign tumor of the colon. In the rectum such a tumor can become quite large, secreting copious mucus material that can be mistaken for diarrhea. Sometimes there are serious losses of sodium and potassium, and some of these benign tumors may become malignant. When a villus adenoma is identified by a colon examination, it should be removed, which will cure the "diarrhea."

Occasionally, a patient may deliberately induce diarrhea with laxatives in a misguided effort to lose weight. When done surreptitiously and without explanation, such laxative abuse is called the *Munchausen syndrome* after the mythical German teller of tall tales, Baron von Munchausen.

Finally, in some cases of persistent diarrhea, repeated investigations fail to reveal a cause, yet spontaneous improvement occurs months or years later. In such instances, the cause remains a mystery.

Investigations

It is important to determine the nature of a patient's diarrhea. The greater the persistence of the diarrhea, the more important it is to conduct investigations. The Bristol Stool Form Scale can help doctors and patients confirm that diarrhea is truly present (figure 6-1). The *Rome III* authors recommend that chronic diarrhea investigation include an erythrocyte sedimentation rate (or

C-reactive protein), hemoglobin (blood count), and serum potassium and albumin levels. When two or more of these four tests are abnormal, a cause for the diarrhea is likely to be found. It is prudent to visualize and biopsy the colonic mucosa by sigmoidoscopy or, preferably, colonoscopy in order to detect IBD, microscopic colitis, villus adenoma or laxative-induced melanosis coli. Steatorrhea is detected through a three-day collection of stool for analysis. This collection includes estimating a twenty-four-hour stool weight; values of 500 grams or more increase suspicion of an organic explanation for the diarrhea. Other tests should be done according to the patient's history and circumstances.

The investigations required to exclude all of the above conditions are many and complex. However, in most Western patients, celiac disease, IBD, and the inadvertent or deliberate ingestion of laxative substances are the most important to consider. The clinical history may suggest others, such as giardiasis in travelers and campers, lactose malabsorption in milk-ingesting people of non-European ancestry, villous adenoma if the diarrhea is clear mucous, and the use of certain medications, especially by the elderly.

What Causes Functional Diarrhea?

As expected, colonic transit is fast in functional diarrhea, but physiologic testing demonstrates little that is unique compared to the known causes of diarrhea or IBS with diarrhea. Possible mechanisms include chronic infection by a yet-to-be-discovered pathogen such as a slow virus, or a tuberculosis-like organism, reduced intestinal mucosal enzymes and absorptive capability following an acute infection, or continued unconscious or covert use of a laxative. Occasionally, the latter phenomenon is discovered by accident. There are few data regarding the psychological state of those with functional diarrhea. Although rapid gut transit is associated with anxiety, it is uncertain if this is cause, effect, or coincidence.

After assessment, a few patients will be determined to have truly functional diarrhea. The diarrhea may be difficult to manage and, unlike the usual diagnostic confidence seen with IBS or functional constipation, functional diarrhea may in time disclose a cause. Therefore, continued diagnostic vigilance is prudent.

Conclusion

Functional diarrhea is characterized by painless, frequent, persistent, loose, watery stools for at least six months and may be found eventually to have one of many causes. Therefore, a careful history and examination are essential to determine which of many tests must be undertaken to diagnose or exclude several diseases. Depending upon circumstances, the most important of these are overt or surreptitious ingestion of food or drugs with laxative properties, lactose intolerance, celiac disease, IBD, and chronic infection with giardiasis. Although all of the functional disorders need follow-up, encouragement, and symptomatic treatment, people with functional diarrhea especially need regular review to detect any new manifestations of disease.

Sources

Afzalpurkar RG, Schiller LR, Little KH, Santangelo WC, Fortran JS. The self-limited nature of chronic idiopathic diarrhoea. *New Engl J Med.* 1992;327:1849-1852.

Bertomeu A, Ros E, Barragan V, Sachje L, Navarro S. Chronic diarrhoea with normal stool and colonic examinations: organic or functional? *J Clin Gastroenterol.* 1991;13:531-536.

Cash BD, Schoenfeld P, Chey WD. The utility of diagnostic tests in irritable bowel syndrome patients: a systematic review. *Am J Gastroenterol.* 2002;97(11):2812-2819.

Drossman DA, Li Z, Andruzzi E, Temple R, Talley NJ, Thompson WG, Whitehead WE, Janssens J, Funch-Jensen P, Corrazziari E, et al. U.S. householder survey of functional gastrointestinal disorders: prevalence, sociodemography, and health impact. *Dig Dis Sci.* 1993;38:1569-1580.

Longstreth GF, Thompson WG, Chey WD, Houghton LA, Mearin F, Spiller RC. Functional bowel disorders. *Gastroenterology.* 2006;130(5):1480-1491.

9 Functional Dyspepsia (Nonulcer Dyspepsia)

> *Dyspepsia [is] a symptom or set of symptoms that . . . originate from the gastroduodenal region. The . . . symptoms are postprandial fullness, early satiation, and epigastric pain or epigastric burning.*
>
> *Functional dyspepsia . . . [consists of] one or more dyspepsia symptoms that . . . originate from the gastroduodenal region [without] any organic, systemic, or metabolic disease . . . to explain [them].*
>
> —Rome III: The Functional Gastrointestinal Disorders

Introduction

Of all the functional gastrointestinal disorders (FGIDs), functional dyspepsia has proven the most difficult to define, and for which to develop precise symptom criteria. There are many putative causes of dyspepsia, and yet the stomach and duodenum appear normal. The Rome working teams have striven to identify the more likely causes through the creation of symptom subgroups. However, as yet no subgroup can be reliably associated with any specific gastroduodenal abnormality. Thus, clinician and patient are faced with the challenges posed in the above definitions: to identify the dyspepsia symptoms, to rule out any known cause (most likely a peptic ulcer) and, when none is found, determine how best to manage the symptoms.

Background

In the nineteenth and early twentieth centuries, upper abdominal pain that occurred regularly after meals very often suggested that there was a peptic ulcer in the stomach or duodenum. However, as diagnostic and surgical techniques developed, it was discovered that many people with such symptoms had no ulcer after all. Such people were said to have "nonulcer" dyspepsia. Originally thought to be due to stomach inflammation called gastritis, it became clear that the symptoms commonly occurred in people with no anatomic abnormality of the stomach or duodenum. Observers noticed that dyspepsia embraced a number of symptoms, including epigastric pain, postmeal fullness, early satiety, bloating, burning, and others (table 9-1).

To try to understand the underlying mechanisms of nonulcer dyspepsia, earlier Rome working teams proposed subgroups: *reflux-like, ulcer-like* and *dysmotility-like* dyspepsia. This division grew from the belief that these subgroups respectively were due to gastroesophageal reflux, excess stomach acid that would respond to acid-lowering drugs, and disordered stomach-emptying that might be corrected by prokinetic drugs. Symptoms thought to be consistent with these abnormalities were the basis for this subgrouping. However, these symptom-based subgroups were found to have little relationship with the putative physiological abnormalities, and proved to be of little practical use. Reflux-like dyspepsia is indistinguishable from heartburn that is due to gastroesophageal reflux disease (GERD). The burning pain linked to ulcer-like dyspepsia and the fullness and satiety of dysmotility-like dyspepsia are unreliable indicators of any underlying acid or motor disorder. Moreover, they fail to indicate effective treatment.

The *Rome III* working team believes that this classification is unhelpful for research as well. Reflux-like dyspepsia is simply heartburn. The team proposes two new symptom-based subgroups; the *postprandial distress syndrome* (PDS), which is the sensation of discomfort or fullness or early satiety after a meal, and the *epigastric pain syndrome* (EPS), which is upper abdominal pain or burning that is not necessarily related to eating. These distinctive subgroups are based on presumed differences in the underlying pathophysiology and are roughly similar to motility-like and ulcer-like in the previous iteration.

Diagnosis
How is Dyspepsia Recognised?

Dyspepsia is difficult to define. Earlier versions describe it as pain or discomfort centered in the upper abdomen, and some insisted that it be meal-related. However, dyspeptic symptoms are several and diverse, and require a more comprehensive definition. The symptoms described in table 9-1 range from epigastric pain, through fullness and satiety, to bloating, nausea, and vomiting. They may or may not be associated with eating. The current definition of functional dyspepsia includes one or more of (1) bothersome postprandial fullness, (2) early satiety, (3) epigastric pain, or (4) epigastric burning that likely originates from the gastroduodenal region. As with other FGIDs there must be no organic, systemic, or metabolic disease to explain the symptoms.

In a dyspeptic patient it is impossible by history alone to exclude common diseases of the gastroduodenum such as peptic ulcer; some investigation is necessary. This usually includes an endoscopic examination of the esophagus, stomach, and duodenum. Dyspeptic patients are either "uninvestigated" or

Table 9-1. Dyspeptic Symptoms and Their Definition

Symptom	Definition
Postprandial fullness	An unpleasant sensation of prolonged persistence of food in the stomach
Early satiation	A feeling that the stomach is overfilled soon after starting to eat, out of proportion to the size of the meal being eaten, so that the meal cannot be finished. Previously, the term "early satiety" was used, but *satiation* is the correct term for the disappearance of appetite during food ingestion.
Epigastric pain	*Epigastric* describes the region between the umbilicus and the lower end of the sternum, bordered by the midclavicular lines. Pain is a subjective, unpleasant sensation; some patients feel damage is occurring. Epigastric pain may or may not have a burning quality. Other symptoms may be extremely bothersome without being interpreted as pain.
Epigastric burning	Burning refers to an unpleasant subjective sensation of heat. As with heartburn, epigastric burning may be due to gastroesophageal reflux.
Bloating in the upper abdomen	An unpleasant sensation of tightness located in the epigastrium; it should be distinguished from visible abdominal distension
Nausea	Queasiness or sick sensation; a feeling of the need to vomit
Vomiting	Forceful oral expulsion of gastric contents associated with contraction of the abdominal and chest wall muscles. It is usually preceded by and associated with retching, repetitive contractions of the abdominal wall.
Belching	Venting of air from the stomach or the esophagus

Adapted from *Rome III: The Functional Gastrointestinal Disorders*, p. 422

"investigated." This difference is important when interpreting prevalence or treatment studies because these two groups of dyspeptic patients yield vastly different results. Only in the investigated group is it possible to separate organic from functional dyspepsia. Thus, dyspepsia invariably requires a negative test to establish a functional diagnosis.

The *Rome III* criteria are shown in table 9-2. The criteria capture the dyspeptic features explained in the previous paragraphs and listed in table 9-1: at least one of bothersome postprandial fullness, early satiation, epigastric pain, or burning. Unlike many other FGIDs, the criteria require a test result—a negative upper gastrointestinal endoscopy. To exclude past or transient illness, the symptoms must be current during the past three months and present for

Table 9-2. Diagnostic Criteria for Functional Dyspepsia

Must include
1. One or more of the following:
   a. Bothersome postprandial fullness
   b. Early satiation
   c. Epigastric pain
   d. Epigastric burning

AND

2. No evidence of structural disease (including at upper endoscopy) that is likely to explain the symptoms

* Criteria fulfilled for the last three months with symptom onset at least six months prior to diagnosis
Rome III: The Functional Gastrointestinal Disorders, p. 427
[For the criteria for the proposed dyspepsia subtypes, please refer to appendix A.]

as long as six months. Unlike previous versions of the diagnostic criteria for functional dyspepsia, heartburn and irritable bowel syndrome (IBS) may coexist with it—a sensible improvement.

The heterogeneity of the symptoms and the variety of proposed causes prompted many attempts to subdivide dyspepsia to more homogeneous entities. Because neither research nor clinical responses now support the prior separation of endoscopy-negative functional dyspepsia patients into "motility-like" and "ulcer-like," the *Rome III* authors propose a different subdivision. Many symptoms such as fullness and satiety are meal-related and are now considered to characterize PDS. When the dyspepsia is localized in the upper abdomen, is intermittent, is not relieved by defecation or flatus, and is not severe and episodic-like pain from inflammation of the pancreas or obstruction of the bile ducts, it is subgrouped as EPS. It is now up to clinical scientists to discover if PDS and EPS have unique pathophysiologies. While the two syndromes may both be present in a single patient, other individuals who fulfill the functional dyspepsia criteria fit neither subgroup. Since PDS and EPS are as yet of unproven value to clinicians and patients, this chapter will concentrate on the diagnosis and putative causes of functional dyspepsia as a whole. Diagnostic criteria for the subgroups are listed in appendix A.

Epidemiology

Because of the several successive definitions and groupings of dyspepsia, published prevalences vary. Using the *Rome II* definition, the prevalence is less than 2% of adults, predominantly females. However, such data refer to "uninvestigated dyspepsia," which includes an unknown number of people with a structural disease. Moreover, the *Rome II* definition excludes IBS and heartburn, so that many dyspeptics are not counted. It is expected that the new criteria will prove to be more accurate, especially if structural disease can be practically excluded (difficult to do in a survey!). The rapid decline in peptic ulcer disease means that in future a greater proportion of dyspeptics will be found to be functional. Meanwhile, dyspepsia's true prevalence remains uncertain.

Other Diagnoses to Consider

The diagnosis of functional dyspepsia is made through recognition of the chronic dyspeptic symptoms believed to emanate from the gastroduodenum (table 9-1). The diagnostic criteria and use of alarm symptoms (table 5-1) serve as useful guides. Heartburn, which usually implies gastroesophageal reflux, can be identified by burning behind the breastbone that worsens with bending, lying, or lifting and is promptly relieved by antacid drugs. An irritable bowel is suspected if the pain is altered with defecation and accompanied by an erratic bowel habit. Abdominal bloating and belching often accompany dyspepsia. *Angina pectoris* (heart pain) may be felt in the chest during physical effort and is relieved by rest. Occasionally angina is felt in the upper abdomen.

The time-honored cause of dyspepsia is a peptic ulcer in either the stomach or duodenum. However, in developed countries, healthier housing conditions, better personal hygiene, and effective treatment have caused a rapid decline in *Helicobacter pylori* infections, which are the principle cause of peptic ulcers. Hence, among dyspeptic patients the proportion of negative endoscopies is much greater than even fifteen years ago. Nevertheless, peptic ulcer is a potentially dangerous disease that can cause major bleeding and other complications. Because ulcers can be cured with an antibiotic regimen, and dyspeptic symptoms are not specific to any diagnosis, new patients should have prompt endoscopy. As the bacterial cause of ulcers declines, a larger proportion of ulcers are caused by prostaglandin-inhibiting aspirin and nonsteroidal anti-inflammatory drugs (NSAIDs). Indeed, anyone with dyspepsia who is taking such drugs should be urgently examined, and the drugs withdrawn if the underlying condition permits. Such drugs may cause dyspepsia with or without an ulcer.

The importance of the medical history is discussed in chapter 5. A physical examination of the abdomen is mandatory to detect any mass or enlarged organ. Many organs lie in the upper abdomen, and the alert physician will have them in mind when examining a dyspeptic patient. Severe epigastric pain that occurs in periodic attacks will suggest stones that are obstructing the bile or pancreatic ducts. Most acute abdominal disease will necessitate an emergency examination, which is beyond our consideration here. Cancer of the stomach, pancreas, or other upper abdominal organ can cause dyspepsia and eventually great pain, but cancer is also characterized by steady deterioration and alarm symptoms.

Comorbid Disease

In addition to IBS, heartburn, belching, and other FGIDs, psychological and nongut somatic symptoms may coexist with functional dyspepsia. These have not been as extensively studied as in IBS, but they should be sought nonetheless to ensure a suitable biopsychosocial treatment approach.

What Causes Functional Dyspepsia?

Two organic diseases influence thinking about the cause of functional dyspepsia. They are diabetic gastroparesis and peptic ulcer. Both cause dyspepsia and serve as models for dyspepsia research. Gastroparesis (literally stomach paralysis) causes delayed gastric emptying of solids. Because gastroparesis is associated with epigastric distress, postprandial fullness, vomiting, bloating, and early satiety, many people wonder if similar symptoms in functional dyspepsia result from a similar disturbance of gastric physiology. The prior predominance of peptic ulcer among dyspeptics leads others to suspect that gastric acid might yet play a key role. Still others suspect that *Helicobacter pylori* might cause dyspepsia in some people. These hypotheses suggest that some dyspeptics might respond to drugs that improve motility, reduce gastric acid, or eradicate *H. pylori*.

Gastroduodenal Dysmotility

Research demonstrates abnormal gastroduodenal motility among many dyspeptics. Overall, gastric emptying—particularly of solids—seems slow, but there is great overlap with control subjects who have normal gastric emptying. A clear abnormality is seen in only a few patients. Other observations include decreased gastric antral contractions and decreased motility responses to nutrients. Poor coordination between the upper and lower parts of the stomach, failure of the stomach to adequately relax (accommodate) after a meal, and abnormal gastric myoelectric activity (stomach-muscle electrical discharges) are also reported. The relationship of such phenomena to symptoms is imprecise, but they are most commonly found in women with fullness, nausea, and vomiting. Patients who present with such phenomema might best fit the PDS subgroup. This idea underpins the use of prokinetic drugs to improve gastric emptying or drugs that relax the stomach to allow it to accommodate a meal. Some clinical trials appear to support this notion, but it is premature to assume that dysmotility causes dyspepsia in some people. If it does, how can doctors clinically identify them?

Gastric Acid Secretion

The stomach's resting secretion of hydrochloric acid is normal in functional dyspepsia, but in some patients the lining of the stomach or duodenum (mucosa) may have increased sensitivity to acid. Powerful inhibitors of acid secretion benefit some of these patients, but in the trials that demonstrate this, it is uncertain whether heartburn (which antacid drugs certainly improve) was excluded. Nevertheless, many dyspeptics have symptoms that resemble peptic ulcer, which tempts physicians to try antiulcer drugs. Such patients may be found among those in the EPS subgroup.

Helicobacter pylori, Chronic Gastritis, and Duodenitis

Gastritis and duodenitis mean inflammation of the inner lining or mucosa of the stomach and duodenum. They range from a local infiltration of inflammatory cells that can only be detected by a microscope to overt superficial ulcerations that behave in many ways like peptic ulcer disease. Such inflammation has long been suspected to cause dyspepsia and to be acid-related. However, the response to acid suppression is inconsistent, and most people with mucosal inflammation have no symptoms that are attributable to it. The situation is complicated by the invariable association of *Helicobacter pylori* with a common form of chronic gastritis. In the past, acid suppressants were regularly tried in such cases with disappointing results. Among those *H. pylori*-infected dyspeptic patients with gastritis, one in seventeen will respond to eradication of the organism. Although in the short term this seems too few for eradication to be clinically justified, the possible prevention of a future peptic ulcer and even the rare cancer may make it so.

Gastroduodenal Hypersensitivity

The visceral hypersensitivity hypothesis outlined in chapter 4 is demonstrable in some patients with functional dyspepsia. Compared to normal people and most other dyspeptics, such patients have lower thresholds for pain during experimental distension of a balloon in the stomach or duodenum. Others may be hypersensitive to stomach or duodenal contents, including acid. In addition to pain, there are sometimes reactive changes in stomach motility. It is not yet known whether these phenomena identify a unique group of dyspeptic patients who might be amenable to sensitivity-reducing treatments.

Other Possible Causes

Some investigations suggest an autonomic nervous system dysfunction in functional dyspepsia. A few patients are reported to have abnormal sympathetic or parasympathetic (vagus) nerve activity. Abnormal hormone levels are noted in others, notably of cholecystokinin and somatostatin. As with other FGIDs, dyspepsia is associated with a variety of psychopathological disorders, especially anxiety. It is possible that, via the brain-gut axis, such disorders affect the gut through neural or hormonal mechanisms.

The Bottom Line

While several plausible mechanisms are proposed, none offers a compelling and substantiated explanation of all functional dyspepsia. This is partly because it is difficult to define the disorder precisely, or to reliably separate dyspeptic patients from those suffering from gastroesophageal reflux and other disorders. The plethora of symptoms that are deemed dyspeptic suggests there may be several dyspepsias, hence the efforts to differentiate groups of dyspeptics with presumably unique physiological mechanisms. Identification of these mechanisms would greatly advance our understanding and eventually lead to more precise treatment. The succession of subtyping proposals represents attempts to address the notion of dyspepsia heterogeneity. Meanwhile, for the majority of dyspeptics, the cause of their symptoms is unknown—and therefore "functional."

Conclusion

Two features make functional dyspepsia unique among the FGIDs. First, many dyspeptic symptoms may imply several underlying physiological disorders. Second, the symptoms are often indicative of an organic disease, notably peptic ulcer and NSAID-induced damage to the upper gut. We have seen the importance of identifying functional dyspepsia patients, but symptom criteria have proven difficult to design, perhaps because of dyspepsia's unique attributes. Past and present publication of criteria for subtypes results from the desire to add precision to diagnosis—and to make research and treatment more rational. Currently, functional dyspepsia is divided into the *postprandial distress syndrome* and the *epigastric pain syndrome*. These sensible symptom groupings must now be tested in patients, and it is likely we shall see more and different subtypes in future.

Source

Tack J, Talley NJ, Camilleri M, Holtmann G, Hu P, Malagelada J R, Stanghellini V. Functional gastroduodenal disorders. In: Drossman DA, Corazziari E, Delvaux M, Spiller RC, Talley NJ, Thompson WG, Whitehead WE, eds. *Rome III: The Functional Gastrointestinal Disorders.* McLean, VA: Degnon Associates, Inc.; 2006:419-485.

10 Heartburn, Chest Pain, Dysphagia: The Functional Esophageal Disorders

> *Functional esophageal disorders are represented by chronic symptoms typifying esophageal disease that have no identified structural or metabolic basis.*
> —*Rome III: The Functional Gastrointestinal Disorders*

Introduction

The physiological and psychosocial mechanisms responsible for the functional esophageal disorders are poorly understood. Most esophageal symptoms that are related to the esophagus *do* have a structural basis, and most frequently this consists of reflux of acid stomach contents into the sensitive lower esophagus (gastroesophageal reflux disease or GERD). However, in some patients with heartburn, chest pain, dysphagia, or globus, no abnormality can be detected. Like other functional gastrointestinal disorders (FGIDs), the symptoms of these functional esophageal disorders often overlap one another. They share two characteristics: there is no evidence that gastroesophageal reflux causes the symptoms, and they fail to improve with powerful acid-suppressing drugs.

Functional Heartburn

> *Functional heartburn is . . . episodic retrosternal burning in the absence of gastroesophageal reflux disease, histopathology-based motility disorders, or structural explanations.*
> — *Rome III: The Functional Gastrointestinal Disorders*

Twenty percent to forty percent of subjects in Western populations suffer from heartburn. It occurs at least once per week in 15% to 20% of individuals irrespective of sex and age; about a third of them seek medical attention. Functional heartburn probably accounts for one in ten heartburn patients who consult gastroenterologists.

Most heartburn sufferers have reflux of acid gastric contents into the esophagus that coincides with a burning pain behind the breastbone. While some people are found to have a lower esophageal inflammation called esophagitis, most have normal-appearing esophageal mucosa. As indicated in the diagnostic criteria (appendix A), functional heartburn is diagnosed when heartburn occurs without evidence that GERD causes the symptom, and no other microscopic or motility disorder explains it.

As with any case of heartburn, it is important to rule out other chronic recurrent chest disorders. Coronary heart disease pain is typically crushing in nature and may radiate to the left arm or neck. Uncommon under age forty-five, the pain commences with effort and is relieved by rest or by taking a nitroglycerine tablet beneath the tongue. Heartburn, on the other hand, is burning in quality. It is worse when the stomach is full and when the person bends, strains, or lies down. Fatty foods and chocolate worsen it as well. Normally, heartburn is promptly relieved by an antacid such as calcium carbonate (Tums), and is prevented by acid-suppressing drugs, particularly the proton pump inhibitors (PPIs) (see chapter 16). As noted in chapter 9, it is sometimes difficult to distinguish heartburn from dyspepsia. Persistent or severe heartburn—especially if it responds poorly to treatment—should prompt an endoscopy to detect or exclude esophagitis. People with heartburn and no esophagitis may yet be sensitive to refluxed acid. A simple test is to give a short course of PPI therapy. If this relieves heartburn, there must be acid reflux. If heartburn is not substantially improved by PPI therapy the patient is deemed to have *functional heartburn*. Specialists may recommend twenty-four-hour ambulatory pH monitoring, in which an acid-sensing device in the lower esophagus detects reflux through the day's activities and indicates whether it occurs with heartburn episodes.

Thus, patients with functional heartburn have a normal-appearing esophagus, do not improve with PPI therapy, and do not have acid reflux episodes that correlate with the symptom. What then causes the heartburn? Is it possible that reflux of weakly acid gastric contents causes the symptom after all, and the PPI fails to sufficiently raise the pH? Could reflux of other material such as alkaline intestinal fluids, or perhaps even esophageal distension, be at fault? Are there esophageal motor and psychological influences? The visceral hypersensitivity hypothesis may explain why functional heartburn patients experience the symptom in response to non-acid-reflux episodes that are insufficient to evoke heartburn in others.

Functional Chest Pain of Presumed Esophageal Origin

Functional chest pain of presumed esophageal origin is characterized by episodes of unexplained midline chest pain of visceral quality, and therefore potentially of esophageal origin.
  — Rome III: The Functional Gastrointestinal Disorders

From 15% to 30% of coronary angiograms performed in patients with chest pain are normal. In most of these cases, the chest pain is presumed to emanate from the esophagus. If 500,000 coronary angiograms are performed in the United States yearly for chest pain, this functional disorder may be present in 75,000 to 150,000 people per year. Functional chest pain of presumed esophageal origin occurs in young people, but most cases that come to medical attention are among heart attack-prone elderly persons who have a negative cardiac workup.

If someone has chest pain, prompt exclusion of cardiac disease is essential. A medical history does not reliably predict the presence or absence of coronary artery disease. The choice of cardiac investigations is influenced by the patient's age, family history, and risk factors. In most cases an exercise (treadmill) electrocardiogram with or without a thallium scan will detect coronary disease. Older patients will undergo coronary angiography.

When cardiac disease is excluded, an endoscopic examination will find esophagitis in fewer than 20% of patients with chest pain. Ambulatory pH monitoring with analysis of the relationship between symptoms and episodes of esophageal acid reflux is the most sensitive method for identifying reflux as the likely cause of chest pain. About 40% of patients with normal coronary angiograms may have acid-related pain. Treadmill testing during ambulatory pH monitoring may be necessary if the pain is associated with exertion; it could be cardiac, esophageal, or both.

However, the most practical test for an acid-sensitive esophagus is symptom relief during PPI treatment. A therapeutic trial with a PPI is inexpensive and seems as accurate as ambulatory pH monitoring. Other diagnostic tests such as esophageal manometry, ambulatory esophageal manometry, esophageal acid perfusion testing, and esophageal balloon distention studies may help reassure patients and doctors that the symptoms are of esophageal origin, but they seldom alter diagnosis or treatment.

Clinical research discloses abnormal responses to esophageal sensory stimuli and altered esophageal motor behavior in patients with functional chest pain. Patients with unexplained chest pain who do not have reflux develop pain with lesser volumes of intraesophageal balloon distention when compared to asymptomatic controls. Such patients also have increased sensitivity to acid in the esophagus. Great accuracy is achieved by measuring balloon pressure thresholds that provoke the pain. Thus, balloon distention sensitivity is a fairly reliable indicator of functional chest pain of presumed esophageal origin. Acid instillation sensitizes the esophagus in susceptible subjects and induces hypersensitivity to other esophageal stimuli (e.g., balloon distention). Subjects with functional chest pain may develop this hypersensitivity after intermittent stimulation by acid reflux. Bolus entrapment in the esophagus during repeated swallows also may cause pain, as may hot and cold liquids.

As in other FGIDs, the visceral hypersensitivity hypothesis provides a rational and practical explanation for functional chest pain of presumed esophageal origin. The hyperalgesic response is provoked by acid or balloon distension in the esophagus. The brain-gut interconnections that facilitate central nervous system involvement are discussed in chapter 4.

Up to half the subjects with unexplained chest pain, but no esophagitis or increased acid exposure, have esophageal motility abnormalities. These include *nutcracker esophagus* (where the amplitude of esophageal contractions is markedly exaggerated) and *diffuse esophageal spasm*, but a causal relationship of such motility disturbances to pain is difficult to establish. These contraction abnormalities may be epiphenomena; that is, they may be bystanders rather than causes. Perhaps they are markers for unknown mechanisms that do cause the pain.

Psychiatric comorbidity is common in patients with chest pain who are referred for further gastroenterological evaluation and lack conspicuous evidence of reflux disease. The presence of anxiety, depression, panic, neuroticism, and somatization is not surprising in people who have become fearful of heart disease. Noncardiac chest-pain patients display less improvement in pain, more frequent pain episodes, greater social maladjustment, and more anxiety symptoms at one-year follow-up than patients with cardiac disease. On the plus side, such patients are unlikely to suffer heart attacks and cardiac deaths in the ten years following diagnosis.

Functional Dysphagia

The disorder is characterized by a sensation of abnormal bolus transit through the esophageal body.
  —Rome III: The Functional Gastrointestinal Disorders

Unlike the irritable bowel syndrome (IBS), functional dysphagia cannot be diagnosed from the medical history, for dysphagia most likely implies a structural disease, which is sometimes very serious (table 10-1). Therefore, the rule is that this functional disorder can only be diagnosed after a fastidious search for several structural causes. If the diagnosis of dysphagia remains uncertain, a brief therapeutic trial with a high-dose PPI may help identify subtle reflux disease.

Table 10-1. Some Causes of Dysphagia That Must be Ruled Out Before Making a Diagnosis of Functional Dysphagia

Cancer of the esophagus
Achalasia
Schatzki's ring
Esophageal stricture
Radiation stricture
Severe esophagitis
Enlarged heart compressing the esophagus
Chest mass: cancer, abscess

Dysphagia investigation requires an endoscopy (with biopsy) to identify reflux esophagitis, cancer, or stricture. A barium-swallow esophageal x-ray with videofluoroscopy and a barium-impregnated "food challenge" during fluoroscopy help identify mucosal rings or strictures that may be otherwise overlooked. These investigations may also detect motility disorders. If endoscopy and biopsy are negative and the barium studies show delayed emptying, they should be followed by esophageal manometry.

In many patients with functional dysphagia, manometry testing discloses several nonspecific esophageal motility abnormalities, including intermittent simultaneous contractions, segmental failure of peristalsis, increased peristaltic wave duration or amplitude, or an inadequately relaxing lower esophageal sphincter. These motor abnormalities have no recognized pathology, and do not support or preclude the diagnosis of functional dysphagia. Here again, visceral hypersensitivity is invoked—the hypersensitive esophagus overreacts to various stimuli that produce motility epiphenomena and a sensation of dysphagia.

Globus

Globus is . . . a sense of a lump or retained food bolus or tightness in the throat.
—*Rome III: The Functional Gastrointestinal Disorders*

Globus is a painless "lump in the throat" that many describe as retained food. It is typically felt behind the upper end of the breastbone. Unlike dysphagia, it is unrelated to meals and improves with eating. Up to half of men and women experience it occasionally.

The cause of this benign symptom is unknown, but dysfunction at or near the upper esophageal sphincter is often suspected. In some patients, there may be coexistent gastroesophageal reflux disease and heartburn, but both globus and heartburn are common and there is little evidence for a causal relationship. Globus may occur with an emotional experience, but is not linked to any psychological disorder.

Diagnosis is made from the patient's description. Confidence in a globus diagnosis is increased if the patient is young and has had the symptoms for several years. There must be no pain, and no difficulty swallowing. Without accompanying symptoms or physical findings in the mouth, throat, and adjacent neck, no tests are required.

Conclusion

Heartburn, chest pain, and dysphagia may indicate serious disease. Respectively, esophagitis, coronary heart disease, and the esophageal lesions listed in table 10-1 must be excluded. In each case the absence of disease and symptom relief with powerful stomach acid suppressants is reassuring. When these symptoms occur with neither underlying disease nor improvement with PPIs, they are said to be functional. Globus, a lump in the throat, has no sinister implications, but nonetheless can be worrisome and annoying.

Source
Galmiche JP, Clouse RE, Bálint A, Cook IJ, Kahrilas PJ, Paterson WG, Smout AJPM. Functional esophageal disorders. In: Drossman DA, Corazziari E, Delvaux M, Spiller RC, Talley NJ, Thompson WG, Whitehead WE, eds. *Rome III: The Functional Gastrointestinal Disorders*. McLean, VA: Degnon Associates, Inc.; 2006:369-417.

11 Incontinence, Anal Pain, Defecation Disorders: The Functional Anorectal Disorders

Introduction

Unlike other functional gastrointestinal disorders (FGIDs), diagnosis of some functional anorectal disorders is assisted by physiological tests as well as the careful assessment of symptoms. Functional fecal incontinence and defecation disorders are better understood using the sophisticated tools that characterize anorectal structure and function. More than merely excluding other diseases, these tests help define the disorders. Moreover, these tests may reveal disturbances of anorectal structure and/or function in patients who were hitherto considered to have a functional disorder. Uniquely, anal physiological measurements are included in the *Rome III* criteria for dyssynergic defecation, discussed under "Functional Defecation Disorders" below.

The distinction between "organic" and "functional" anorectal disorders is often blurred for the following reasons: the relationship between structural abnormalities and anorectal symptoms is often obscure; structural abnormalities are observed in asymptomatic subjects; lesions such as rectal prolapse or pudendal nerve injury may be the result rather than the cause of repeated straining and; a patient may have both a structural and a functional disturbance such as diarrhea and incontinence. Despite this structural/functional ambiguity, the functional anorectal disorders appear to result from abnormal function of normally innervated and structurally intact anorectal and pelvic floor muscles.

Functional Fecal Incontinence

Fecal incontinence is recurrent uncontrolled passage of fecal material for at least three months.
 —Rome III: The Functional Gastrointestinal Disorders

The diagnosis of functional incontinence requires uncontrolled passage of fecal material by a person who is developmentally more than four years of

Table 11-1. Common Causes of Fecal Incontinence

Anal sphincter weakness
Traumatic: obstetric, surgical (hemorrhoidectomy, sphincterotomy)
Nontraumatic: scleroderma, internal sphincter degeneration of unknown cause

Neuropathy
Peripheral (pelvic nerve) or generalized (diabetes mellitus)

Disturbances of pelvic floor
Rectal prolapse, descending perineum syndrome

Inflammatory conditions
Radiation proctitis, Crohn's disease, ulcerative colitis

Central nervous system disorders
Dementia, stroke, brain tumor, multiple sclerosis, spinal cord lesion

Diarrhea
Irritable bowel syndrome, postcholecystectomy diarrhea

Other
Fecal retention with overflow, behavioral disorders with deliberate retention of stool (*encopresis* in children)

Adapted from *Rome III: The Functional Gastrointestinal Disorders*, p.654.

age, with one or more of the following: abnormally functioning anal muscles; minor abnormalities in sphincter structure or nerve control; constipation with retention of stool in the rectum; diarrhea; or psychological disturbance. Involuntary passing of flatus alone does not qualify as functional fecal incontinence even though patients may be distressed by it. Clear mucus secretions leaking from the anus may originate from a villous tumor or rectal prolapse and must be distinguished from leaking feces. Nocturnal incontinence is uncommon and is most frequently encountered in patients with systemic conditions such as diabetes or scleroderma. Dementia or behavioral problems sometimes lead to willful soiling or social indifference to continence. Incontinence is not considered functional if there is a central, peripheral, or local nervous abnormality, or if the anus is damaged by disease or injury. Table 11-1 lists conditions that cause fecal incontinence and must be excluded before functional fecal incontinence can be diagnosed.

Many patients are terrified by the possibility and unpredictability of incontinence episodes. Therefore, it is important to understand the incontinent patient's coping behavior, self-perception, embarrassment, and day-to-day limitations, including restricted ability to leave the house and socialize.

The clinical history should establish whether fecal incontinence is associated with diarrhea, constipation, or fecal retention. It should also reveal any clues to the presence of sphincter muscle injuries (e.g., obstetrical tears, fistulous disease due to Crohn's, rectal resection, or radiation) or abnormal enervation (e.g., diabetes mellitus, spinal cord injury, or stroke). Some patients have an exaggerated urge to defecate before leaking occurs but cannot reach the toilet in time; others leak stool unawares or passively. This distinction between urge and passive incontinence helps identify the cause. Urge incontinence suggests external anal sphincter weakness, reduced rectal capacity, or rectal hypersensitivity. Passive incontinence suggests injury to the internal anal sphincter or decreased rectal sensitivity. Testing is needed to verify these clues.

Fecal continence is maintained by several factors, including the pelvic floor muscles, rectal curves, transverse rectal folds, rectoanal sensation, and rectal relaxation pending defecation (figure 3-5). Diarrhea or, paradoxically, fecal impaction may overcome these normal mechanisms, but anal sphincter weakness is the most frequently identified abnormality in incontinent patients. Internal anal sphincter dysfunction may be characterized by exaggerated spontaneous relaxation. External anal sphincter weakness may result from sphincter damage or impaired enervation, sometimes caused by childbirth. The levator ani and puborectalis muscles may also function abnormally in fecal incontinence.

Because of the systemic causes of incontinence, the physical examination should be comprehensive. A rectal examination may detect local disease, fecal impaction, decreased anal sensation, reduced anal squeeze, or weakened resting anal pressure. The puborectalis muscle normally should contract in concert with the anal sphincter. A rectal prolapse or excessive perineal (pelvic floor) descent may best be detected with the patient sitting on a commode. Endoscopic examination of the rectum and sigmoid colon will discover obvious structural abnormalities.

Anorectal manometry measures anorectal function by employing a catheter assembly that includes a balloon positioned in the rectum and pressure transducers within the anal canal (see appendix B). Rectal distention induces reflex relaxation of the internal anal sphincter. It is perceived as a sensation of rectal fullness, as if the rectum were uncomfortably full of flatus or feces. If defecation is inconvenient, the desire to defecate prompts voluntary contraction of the external sphincter. As the rectum accommodates more stool, the desire wanes together with the sense of urgency. Sphincter pressures alone do not always distinguish continent from incontinent subjects. Reduced rectal sensation allows stool to enter the anal canal, and perhaps leak before the external sphincter contracts. Anorectal manometry may be followed by biofeedback training for fecal incontinence or pelvic floor dyssynergia.

The anus may also be examined by anal ultrasound. This technique may show a surgically correctable sphincter muscle defect. Sphincter and pelvic floor function can be further assessed in real time by using x-ray fluoroscopy to observe the anorectum expelling barium (defecography). Magnetic resonance imaging and certain neurophysiologic tests complete the assessment.

Execution and interpretation of these tests require a specialist at a properly equipped medical center.

Functional Anorectal Pain

There are two types of functional anorectal pain: *chronic proctalgia* (steady pain) and *proctalgia fugax* (fleeting pain). They are distinguished from one another by duration (hours or days of constant pain for chronic proctalgia vs. seconds or minutes for proctalgia fugax), *frequency* (constant or frequent vs. infrequent), and quality of pain (dull pain or urgency vs. sharp pain). There is overlap between these two painful and sometimes embarrassing conditions, but they are likely to have different physiological mechanisms.

Chronic Proctalgia

Chronic proctalgia is a long-lasting, vague, dull ache or pressure sensation high in the rectum and is often worse when sitting than when standing or lying. When digital rectal examination discovers tightly contracted levator ani muscles and tenderness, chronic proctalgia is called the *levator ani syndrome*. If this is not found and the patient does not fit the description for the much briefer proctalgia fugax, the patient is said to have *unspecified functional anorectal pain*.

Evaluation includes sigmoidoscopy and imaging studies such as ultrasonography, pelvic computed tomography, or magnetic resonance imaging to exclude alternative diseases. The pathophysiology of functional anorectal pain is poorly understood, but the levator ani syndrome may result from overly contracted pelvic floor muscles and higher-than-normal anal resting pressures. It is characterized by tenderness of the puborectalis and periods of chronic or recurrent rectal pain or ache lasting more than twenty minutes. No observable local disease is found. During puborectalis muscle palpation in the levator ani syndrome, the tenderness is usually left-sided; massage may elicit the characteristic discomfort. In unspecifed functional anorectal pain the puborectalis is not tender.

Proctalgia Fugax

This is a sudden, severe pain in the anal area lasting several seconds to as long as thirty minutes, and then disappearing completely. Only 10% of patients report that the pain lasts more than five minutes. These attacks of anal pain are infrequent, typically occurring less than five times per year. People with proctalgia fugax describe the pain is "cramping," "gnawing," "aching," or "stabbing" and it may range from uncomfortable to unbearable. At least half of those who experience proctalgia fugax must interrupt their normal activities or are awakened during an attack.

Up to 18% of men and women experience these otherwise harmless attacks; they are so brief that most patients do not report them to a doctor. The cause of these unpredictable episodes is unknown, but spasm or cramping of the anal sphincters or pelvic floor muscles are suspect. As with the other FGIDs, care should be taken not to miss other causes of anal pain such as prostatitis or anal fissure. Nevertheless, the diagnosis is usually made from the patient's description of the pain, its fleeting occurrence, and its independence of defecation, urination, or intercourse.

Functional Defecation Disorders

Functional constipation, discussed in chapter 7, may be due to slow colon transit or difficulty in emptying stool from the rectum (outlet delay), but these are usually mild and transit time is within the normal range. However, patients with *functional defecation disorders* have either slow transit or outlet delay—or both. Paradoxical contraction or inadequate relaxation of the pelvic floor muscles or inadequate contraction of the abdominal wall muscles during attempted defecation is called *dyssynergic defecation*. However, before functional outlet-delay can be diagnosed, structural lesions such as a stricture from scar tissue, rectocele, or rectal prolapse must be ruled out.

Investigation for defecation disorders is required when constipation stubbornly persists after exhaustive treatments, especially if the intestinal transit time is prolonged. The readily available and inexpensive radiopaque marker test described in chapter 7 can be used to measure transit through the whole gut. Delay of the ingested markers in the sigmoid colon and rectum may suggest dyssynergia, but this can also occur with slow-transit constipation.

Symptoms thought to be associated with functional defecation disorders include straining, feeling of incomplete evacuation after defecation, digital facilitation of defecation, and a sensation of trouble letting go when attempting to defecate. However, these do not consistently distinguish patients with functional constipation from those with functional defecation disorders. The criteria for these disorders must rely on those of functional constipation (table 7-1) plus abnormal physiological tests.

Dyssynergic Defecation

In a patient with chronic constipation, the diagnosis of dyssynergic defecation is based on inappropriate pelvic floor contraction or less than 20% relaxation of resting sphincter pressure during attempted defecation. This functional disorder is unique in that the *Rome III* criteria include an abnormal physiologic measurement. However, dyssynergic defecation patterns occur in some "normal" people under certain circumstances and do not necessarily correlate with symptoms. For example, apparent dyssynergy results from fear of passing stool during a physical examination.

The time required to expel balloons filled with water or air from the rectum is a useful screening test for a functional defecation disorder, but it does not establish the mechanism. The balloon expulsion test may also be abnormal in patients with mechanical causes of outlet delay. For this test a patient sits on a commode chair and strains, while manometric changes in rectal and anal pressures are recorded in a manner similar to those for fecal incontinence. During attempts to defecate there is a paradoxical contraction, or failure of relaxation, of the pelvic floor, including the puborectalis muscle.

Defecography is a dynamic radiological technique to evaluate the rectum and pelvic floor during attempted defecation. Briefly, barium sulfate that is thickened to the consistency of soft stool is injected into the rectum. X-ray or videofluoroscopy characterizes pelvic floor function while the patient is resting and while straining to defecate. This test can detect structural abnormalities including rectocele, enterocele, intussusception, rectal prolapse, and megarectum. In addition, defecography can assess the anorectal angle at rest and during straining, perineal descent, anal diameter, indentation of the contracted puborectalis, and degree of rectal emptying. However, typical manometry findings and delayed balloon expulsion are usually sufficient to diagnose a functional defecation disorder in a patient who has no relevant structural disease.

Inadequate Defecatory Propulsion

A functional defecation disorder may also be caused by inadequate propulsive forces, characterized by a decreased or absent intrarectal pressure during attempted defecation. This may be clinically indistinguishable from, or may occur with, dyssynergic defecation. Rarely, extreme failure of defecatory propulsion results from damaged colonic nerves or muscle (e.g., spinal cord injury or Lou Gherig disease).

Conclusion

No other functional disorders can generate more embarrassment and impaired quality of life than the defecation disorders. Incontinence, rectal pain, and the inability to defecate are life challenges for the patient and management challenges for the therapist. The first step is a thorough clinical assessment to be sure no remedial contributing disease is overlooked. Rational management cannot be contemplated until a precise diagnosis is established. Diagnosis is the beginning of treatment and a means to restore a patient's confidence and self respect.

Source

Wald A, Bharucha AE, Enck P, Rao S. Functional anorectal disorders. In: Drossman DA, Corazziari E, Delvaux M, Spiller RC, Talley NJ, Thompson WG, Whitehead WE, eds. *Rome III: The Functional Gastrointestinal Disorders*. McLean, VA: Degnon Associates Inc.; 2006: 639-685.

12 Belching, Bloating, Pain, and the Other Functional Gastrointestinal Disorders

Introduction

The remaining functional gastrointestinal disorders (FGIDs) are summarized here. Little is known about some of them, and for some there is no specific treatment. Others, such as bloating and chronic pain, may be very troublesome. The functional biliary disorders are complex, controversial in their management, and require special testing. Diagnostic criteria for these disorders appear in appendix A.

Belching Disorders

People normally swallow air while eating and drinking. Distention of the stomach with air triggers transient lower esophageal sphincter (LES) relaxations to allow the air to be vented. Next, the upper esophageal sphincter relaxes in response to esophageal distension. Approximately 18 ml of air is ingested with a liquid swallow, and up to four belches per hour normally follow a meal. Hence, belching is a normal phenomenon and can only be considered a disorder when it becomes troublesome.

Aerophagia

Aerophagia is air swallowing that can lead to excessive belching. It is diagnosed by observing a patient's excessive, yet not always obvious, air gulping. To swallow air, a negative pressure is generated within the esophagus by expanding the chest with the glottis (windpipe) closed, thereby sucking air in. The subsequent belch is characterized by a rapid in-and-out esophageal flow of air that usually fails to reach the stomach. This "supragastric belching," unlike normal gastric belching, requires neither gastric distension nor transient LES relaxation.

When aerophagia is disclosed through a careful history and observation, no investigation is required. Sometimes esophageal pH monitoring demonstrates a temporal association between belching and acid reflux events. Since excessive belching may accompany gastroesophageal reflux disease, a trial of acid suppression therapy with a proton pump inhibitor may break the reflux-aerophagia-belch cycle. A patient with functional dyspepsia may be sensitive to gastric distension and deliberately belch to relieve the symptoms. Emotion can increase spontaneous swallowing in some healthy people. While psychological factors may be important in aerophagia, there is no evidence of psychopathology.

Unspecified Excessive Belching
Unspecified excessive belching, like aerophagia, is "troublesome repetitive belching at least several times a week," but air swallowing is not observed.

Nausea and Vomiting Disorders
Nausea is an unpleasant sensation of an imminent need to vomit and is experienced in the upper abdomen or throat. Vomiting is the forceful oral expulsion of gastric or intestinal contents accompanied by contraction of abdominal and chest wall muscles. Nausea is common and has many possible causes. It sometimes occurs with queasiness, epigastric discomfort, sweating, lightheadedness, fatigue, and emotional symptoms.

Chronic Idiopathic Nausea
Chronic idiopathic nausea consists of bothersome nausea at least several times per week, usually unassociated with vomiting. To be functional, there must be no structural explanation or drug use, notably cannabis.

Functional Vomiting
Unexplained (functional) vomiting is uncommon, and distinct from the vomiting that occasionally occurs with functional dyspepsia. The term *psychogenic vomiting* is now abandoned. Population-based data using *Rome II* criteria suggest that functional vomiting occurs in about .04% of adults. Vomiting differs from regurgitation and rumination. *Regurgitation* describes ingested food returning to the mouth with no abdominal or chest muscle contraction. *Rumination* is the repeated voluntary regurgitation of food.

Many possible causes of nausea and vomiting are listed in table 12-1. Fortunately, most can be confidently excluded by a careful history, physical examination, and use of the diagnostic criteria and alarm symptoms.

Cyclic Vomiting Syndrome (CVS)
CVS is characterized by episodes of vomiting with a stereotypical onset and duration and varying asymptomatic intervals of no vomiting. It occurs at all ages, but is rare in adults. Many children with cyclic vomiting have a family history of migraine headaches. Episodes last a few days and may be linked to menses or precipitated by pregnancy. Adult patients have about four vomiting cycles per year compared to twelve per year in children.

Table 12-1. Differential Diagnosis of Nausea and Vomiting (Categories with Examples)

Disorders of the gut and peritoneum
  Mechanical obstruction
    Gastric outlet or small-bowel obstruction
  Functional gastrointestinal disorders
    Functional dyspepsia, irritable bowel syndrome
  Organic gastrointestinal disorders
    Gastroparesis, chronic intestinal pseudoobstruction
  Pancreatic cancer
  Inflammatory abdominal disease
    Cholecystitis, pancreatitis

Medications and toxic substances
  Cancer chemotherapy
  Analgesics
    Aspirin, nonsteroidal antiinflammatory drugs
  Cardiovascular medications
    Digoxin, antiarrhythmics
  Hormonal preparations/therapies
    Oral antidiabetics, contraceptives
  Antibiotics/antivirals
    Erythromycin, acyclovir
  Gastrointestinal medications
    Sulfasalazine, azathioprine
  Central nervous system active medications
    Narcotics, anti-Parkinson drugs

continues

Rumination Syndrome in Adults

Ruminant animals such as sheep, cattle, and goats have stomachs with several chambers. Ingested food in the upper chamber regurgitates into the mouth by coordinated, retrograde peristalsis while the LES relaxes. The animals then rechew and reswallow the regurgitated food. This process aids digestion by reducing particle size and enhancing acid exposure. In humans, rumination is characterized by repetitive, effortless regurgitation of ingested food into the mouth followed by rechewing and reswallowing. It was initially described in infants and the developmentally disabled, but is observed uncommonly in men and women of all ages and intelligence. Sometimes regurgitation is reported to the doctor by a relative who is disgusted by its occurrence at dinner.

The available physiological evidence suggests that this syndrome occurs when there is paradoxical relaxation of the lower esophageal sphincter in the presence of increased intra-abdominal pressure, or relaxation of the dia-

Table 12-1 continued. Differential Diagnosis of Nausea and Vomiting (Categories with Examples)

Medications and toxic substances
Antiasthmatics
Theophylline
Ethanol abuse
Hypervitaminosis

Infections
Gastrointestinal: viral or bacterial gastroenteritis
Nongastrointestinal: otitis media (middle ear infection)

Endocrine/metabolic disorders
Pregnancy, diabetic ketoacidosis

After general anesthetic

CNS disorders
Migraine
Increased intracranial pressure, cancer, cerebral bleeding
Seizure disorders
Demyelinating disorders
Motion sickness, Meniere's disease

Psychiatric disorders
Psychogenic vomiting, anorexia nervosa

Cardiac disease
Myocardial infarction, congestive heart failure

Starvation

Adapted from *Rome III: The Functional Gastrointestinal Disorders*, p.459-460

---

phragm, which normally exerts a closing pressure on the lower esophagus. Possibly it is a learned behavior.

Ruminating adults are often mistakenly thought to regurgitate because of gastroparesis or gastroesophageal reflux. Rumination must be considered when there is regurgitation, postprandial vomiting (without retching), and weight loss (especially in adolescents). Many ruminants have nausea, heartburn, abdominal discomfort, and bowel dysfunction. The disorder is common in adolescent girls, and with weight loss it may be mistakenly thought to be bulimia or anorexia nervosa. Typical clinical features include the following:

- Repetitive regurgitation of gastric contents within minutes of commencing a meal. Chronic vomiting after meals suggests gastroparesis.
- Rumination is effortless and lasts one to two hours.
- It may be preceded by belching but not by retching or nausea.

- The regurgitant is partially recognizable food, which patients claim has an initial pleasant taste. Some report the regurgitant later becomes sour, acidic, or bitter tasting, which prompts them to cease ruminating.
- Regurgitating patients may decide to swallow or reject the regurgitant, depending upon on the social situation.
- Rumination is typically "meal in, meal out, day in, day out."

Functional Bloating

Bloating is a recurrent sensation of abdominal distension that may or may not be associated with measurable distension but is not part of another functional bowel or gastroduodenal disorder.
—Rome III: The Functional Gastrointestinal Disorders

Abdominal bloating is often viewed as synonymous with abdominal distension, but girth is not always increased. Typically, bloating (with or without increasing girth) worsens as the day progresses and it subsides overnight. Belching, borborygmi (audible bowel sounds), and passage of flatus may accompany bloating, but are not causally related. Bloating often occurs with irritable bowel syndrome (IBS), chronic constipation, dyspepsia, and premenstrual syndrome. Whether as a stand-alone symptom or part of another disorder, bloating is a very common complaint, especially among women.

The normal intestine contains approximately 200 ml of gas, mainly nitrogen, oxygen, hydrogen, carbon dioxide, and methane. Most intestinal nitrogen and oxygen is from swallowed air, while hydrogen, carbon dioxide, and methane result from colonic bacterial fermentation of unabsorbed carbohydrate and protein. The interaction of gastric acid and bicarbonate produces carbon dioxide, but that gas is so rapidly absorbed and exhaled that it contributes little to distension.

Older explanations of bloating include hysteria, excess lumbar lordosis (sagging back), depression of the diaphragm, and voluntary protrusion of the abdomen. More recent hypotheses propose gas accumulation, paradoxical relaxation of the anterior abdominal wall muscles with failure of the diaphragm muscles to relax after eating, thus leading to abdominal protrusion, or sensory nerve dysfunction. These have been called viscerosensory dysfunction. Most bloating research is in IBS or dyspepsia patients, rather than those with bloating alone. Gas retention data on bloating patients vary with the techniques used to measure it. Inert gas washout experiments show similar endogenous gas production and composition in people with and without gas-related complaints. Computed tomography discloses no excess gas in most IBS patients who are experiencing abdominal distension. However, other investigators using radioactive materials find that gas retention in IBS patients exceeds that of healthy volunteers. Probiotics and antibiotics that are designed to reduce bowel gas by altering gut flora fail to improve bloating. Ingestion of psyllium (fermentable fiber), methylcellulose (nonfermentable fiber), bran, and lactulose often increases the sensation. In summary, most evidence suggests that bloating is not solely due to intestinal gas, nor has research revealed any consistent alteration in intestinal transit.

A bloating patient's girth may increase by 12 cm throughout the day. However, gas distension of the abdomen seems an insufficient explanation of the distension that accompanies bloating. Because of expeditious gas transit and evacuation, most healthy volunteers tolerate large gas infusions into the jejunum. Nevertheless, jejunal gas induces more bloating than an equivalent volume of gas in the rectum, and distension is related to the volume. There is little evidence that the abdominal muscles behave uniquely in bloated patients, but there may be altered visceral sensation.

Population surveys associate bloating with depression and other psychological problems. In women with IBS, depression and bloating accompany one another; many report that stress and anxiety exacerbate distension. Despite these data, most people with bloating alone have no psychopathology.

Unspecified Functional Bowel Disorder

Some bowel symptoms that are commonly found in IBS, functional bloating, constipation, or diarrhea either occur alone, or are insufficient to constitute a functional bowel disorder. They are common, but seldom troublesome.

Functional Abdominal Pain Syndrome (FAPS)

Functional abdominal pain syndrome describes continuous, nearly continuous, or frequently recurrent pain localized to the abdomen but poorly related to gut function.
—*Rome III: The Functional Gastrointestinal Disorders*

FAPS describes pain attributed to the abdomen that is poorly related to gut function, associated with some loss of daily activities, and present for at least six months. It is also called "chronic idiopathic abdominal pain" and "chronic functional abdominal pain." The pain is constant, or at least frequently recurring, often with other somatic symptoms. It differs from that of IBS and functional dyspepsia by its poor relationship to eating or defecation. Patients may describe FAPS in emotional terms like "nauseating" or "stabbing like a knife." Often the pain is constant and occurs over a large, imprecise anatomic area. Some maladaptive symptom-related behaviors accompany FAPS (table 12-2), but have little diagnostic value. Depression and anxiety frequently accompany chronic pain. Some psychiatrists would argue that FAPS is not a bowel disorder at all, but rather a somatoform pain disorder, or hypochondriasis.

Physical examination can not establish a diagnosis of FAPS. Nevertheless, examination has several important roles. First, it clarifies pain location and

Table 12-2. Maladaptive Symptom-Related Behaviors in Patients with FAPS

1. Verbally or nonverbally expressed pain intensity may diminish when the patient is distracted and increase when discussing a psychologically distressing issue or during examination.
2. Urgent reporting of intense symptoms is disproportionate to available clinical and laboratory data (e.g., the pain is always rated 10 out of 10).
3. Psychosocial contributors, anxiety, or depression are minimized, denied, or attributed to the pain rather than understandable life circumstances.
4. Tests or exploratory surgery are requested to prove the condition is "organic."
5. Complete relief of symptoms is sought rather than coping with a chronic disorder.
6. Health care-seeking is frequent.
7. Little personal responsibility for self-management is taken and high expectations are placed on the physician.
8. Narcotics are requested.

Adapted from *Rome III: The Functional Gastrointestinal Disorders,* p. 565.

pattern. Physical findings direct the diagnostic workup and occasionally discover an underlying cause, such as abdominal wall pain. The examination also provides an opportunity for the doctor to assess the pain's emotional impact. Despite severe, constant pain an FAPS patient may easily move around the room or onto the examination table. Poor eye contact and other emotional behaviors betray hostility, embarrassment, low self-esteem, mistrust, anxiety, or distress. As with any patient, alarm signs and abnormal physical findings or laboratory results (e.g., anemia, high sedimentation rate, low serum albumin, blood in the stool) should prompt appropriate investigation. When other causes have been ruled out and the criteria are met, a diagnosis of FAPS is probable.

Some FAPS characteristics are listed in table 12-3. Understanding the emotional impact of the pain and performing a physical examination are two essential steps toward providing effective reassurance. In addition, the following psychosocial observations should be addressed:

1. FAPS patients have frequent health care visits for two years or longer for painful complaints and are assigned poorly justified diagnoses such as adhesions or gastroenteritis. Other chronic pain conditions (e.g., fibromyalgia, pelvic pain, headaches, and back pain) often complicate management.
2. The long duration of abdominal pain (average seven years when referred to a pain clinic) entails many exacerbations, visits, and hospitalizations. The circumstances surrounding the first and other

Table 12-3. Characteristics of FAPS Detected During Physical Examination

Feature	Implication
No autonomic arousal	No tachycardia, hypertension, or sweating that are usually seen in acute pain due to structural causes
Abdominal surgical scars	Multiple scars from surgical procedures that were performed for unclear indications, which may suggest the procedures were unneeded
"Closed-eyes sign"	Wincing, closed eyes during abdominal examination contrasts with the fearful eyes-wide-open anticipation of acute structural pain
"Stethoscope sign"	Pain reporting is less when an examiner applies a stethoscope to the painful abdomen than when she purposely palpates it.

Adapted from *Rome III: The Functional Gastrointestinal Disorders*, p. 567

major presentations as well as the current visit are important. These may be fear of serious disease, stress, worsening function, a hidden agenda (seeking narcotics, litigation, disability status, or illness legitimization), or coincident psychiatric disturbance.
3. Previous traumatic events such as emotional, sexual, or physical abuse, death, divorce, and losses due to abortion, stillbirth, or hysterectomy are common and predict a poor outcome.
4. Quality of life and social and employment functioning are revealed by the answers to, "How much is this affecting your life?" or "What would you do differently if you did not have this pain?"
5. Psychiatric diagnoses frequently accompany FAPS. Depression and anxiety are treatable, but personality disorders and substance abuse are less so.
6. Dysfunctional family interactions add to the stress and the illness may be a means to divert conflict. This is apparent when the spouse or parent indulges the patient, assumes undue responsibility, or is the patient's spokesperson.
7. Cultural beliefs complicate management—Asian cultures stigmatize mental difficulties, but Italians and Jews are likely to accept emotional expression.
8. "Catastrophizing" or perceived hopelessness, pessimism, and a sense of poor control over the illness frequently accompany FAPS.

If patient and physician agree that the pain is a chronic "mind-body" disorder with psychosocial contributions to exacerbations, a treatment plan is possible. If the patient's goal is to "find the cause and obtain cure," realistic

The Experience of Pain

- Greatest in acute pain,
- End-organ dominant

  Rx: analgesic

Sensory Discrimination

Affective - Motivational
- Greatest in chronic pain,
- CNS dominant: anxiety

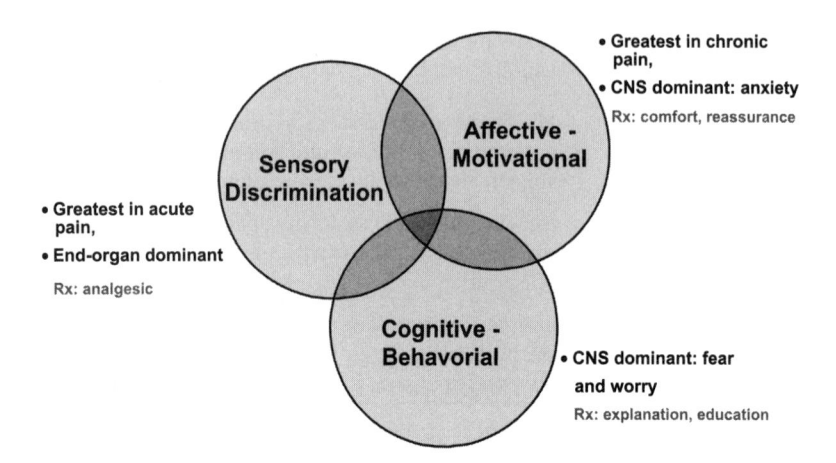

  Rx: comfort, reassurance

Cognitive - Behavorial
- CNS dominant: fear and worry

  Rx: explanation, education

Figure 12-1. Pain has three dimensions. The sensory discriminatory dimension is dominant in acute pain when one has sustained an injury. It is end-organ dependent and "hard-wired" to the brain. The pain sensors in the hurt part transmit to lower centers in the brain, where awareness occurs, and to the cerebral cortex, which localizes and interprets the pain. Pain killers such as codeine may bring relief. The cognitive-behavioral and affective-emotional dimensions are those that embrace fear, worry, and anxiety about the pain. These dimensions are dominant in chronic pain and are central nervous system (CNS)-dominant. Traditional pain killers are less effective in chronic pain.

treatment is difficult. Psychological interventions such as cognitive behavioral treatments may help.

Pain has a sensory-discrimination component, a cognitive-behavioral component, and an affective-motivational component (figure 12-1). The first component is pain that occurs in response to an acute injury. The pain is transmitted from pain receptors in the affected part to the cerebral cortex. This sensory component responds to analgesic drug therapy. However, emotional, cognitive, and affective-motivational factors affect the modulation, and therefore the central recognition of the injury. These are prominent in chronic pain. FAPS symptoms are constant and unrelated to food intake or defecation, which suggests that gut sensory nerves play little part. Moreover, FAPS improvement on low-dose tricyclic antidepressants implies either central or peripheral neuropathic pain. Because it is dominated by central cognitive and emotional influences, chronic pain is less likely to respond to analgesics and may require treatments that are directed to the central nervous system such as antidepressants or psychotherapy. Sometimes, a neuropathic pain results from a nerve injury due to abdominal surgery or childbirth, with continuing sensory input to the spinal cord. However, it is likely that FAPS is more complicated than neuropathic pain and that the central nervous system's role is most important.

FAPS often occurs with anxiety, depression, and somatization, which may alter cognitive or emotional regulation of the pain. Modulating brain mechanisms inhibit and facilitate the pain experience through pathways that originate in the brainstem. These regulate spinal cord nervous excitability and determine how much gut sensation is allowed to reach the brain and therefore consciousness. Descending inhibitory nerves can attenuate pain sensation. Some suggest that patients with chronic pain syndromes, including fibromyalgia and FAPS, may have compromised central pain modulation, or an imbalance between pain facilitation and inhibition. Pain modulation systems originate in prefrontal and cingulate cortical areas of the brain and descend to the brainstem where they control spinal cord excitability and pain sensitivity.

The cerebral cortex is the brain's outer layer and site of the highest neurological and intellectual activity. Could the cortex's connections to brain regions involved in pain modulation and emotion be the basis for the emotional characterizations of pain by FAPS patients? Their beliefs and coping styles include focusing attention on symptoms, "catastrophizing," and denying psychosocial factors. Thus, the cortex, influenced by stress, may alter pain modulation. Using brain imaging techniques, investigators have shown a connection between stress and increased activation in areas of the brain associated with pain activation.

FAPS patients are not malingering. The lack of relationship between bowel activity and pain appears to indicate psychological dysfunction. Psychological well-being and quality of life are more impaired if abdominal pain is associated with other somatic symptoms such as faintness, dizziness, breathlessness, and weakness. FAPS patients with ineffective coping strategies or poor social or family support suffer more pain, more psychological distress, and poorer clinical outcomes.

Functional Gallbladder and Sphincter of Oddi Disorders

The gallbladder (GB) and sphincter of Oddi (SO) regulate bile flow from the liver through the biliary tract into the duodenum (figure 3-4). The flow of pancreatic secretions into the duodenum is similarly regulated. Obstruction of this apparatus may cause intermittent upper abdominal pain, transient elevation of liver function tests (LFTs) and pancreatic enzymes, bile duct dilatation, or pancreatitis. These, especially pancreatitis, require prompt medical attention. There are many causes of such obstruction, most notably gallstones, but functional GB disorder is characterized by bile stasis and pain due to disturbed bile duct motility that causes increased gallbladder pressure. The functional SO disorders encompass abnormal motility of the biliary SO, pancreatic SO, or both, when the gallbladder has been removed. The motility abnormalities of the GB and biliary SO produce pain similar to that of a gallbladder attack due to gallstones (biliary colic), whereas abnormalities of the pancreatic SO cause pain that is similar to that of pancreatitis. The diagnosis of these three entities—functional GB disorder, functional biliary SO disorder, and functional pancreatic SO disorder—depends upon specific symptoms and exclusion of structural causes.

Disorders of the GB and SO share common diagnostic criteria (see appendix A): episodes of pain in the upper abdomen under the right ribs for thirty minutes or more at irregular intervals. The pain builds to a steady level, interrupts activity, and may prompt a visit to a hospital emergency department. It is unrelated to defecation or posture, and is unrelieved by antacids. Pain may awaken one at night, be associated with nausea and vomiting, and be felt in the back or under the right shoulder blade.

Functional gallbladder and sphincter of Oddi disorders are uncommon, and some even question if they exist. Investigation requires highly expert endoscopic retrograde cholangiopancreatography (ERCP) with measurements of duct pressure. These procedures carry a significant risk of pancreatitis.

Functional Gallbladder Disorder

To diagnose this condition, the criteria must be present, the gallbladder must be intact, and the LFTs and the pancreatic enzymes (amylase and lipase) in the blood must be normal. The symptoms of functional GB disorder are similar to those due to gallstones, but far less common. Transabdominal ultrasonography of the upper abdomen is mandatory in patients with biliary symptoms: in functional gallbladder disorder ultrasound should reveal a normal biliary tract and pancreas without evidence of gallstones, sludge, or other disease. Endoscopic ultrasonography is even more accurate. Careful microscopic examination of gallbladder bile obtained at ERCP will detect tiny stones and cholesterol microcrystals that could obstruct the ducts.

Functional Biliary SO Disorder

This disorder is diagnosed if the criteria for disorders of the GB and SO are present and pancreatic enzymes are normal. Only diagnosed in patients whose gallbladder is removed, this uncommon disorder could have been responsible for the organ's removal in the first place. The diagnosis is most convincing if LFTs are transiently abnormal during or after at least two attacks of pain. Biliary SO dysfunction is characterized by motility abnormalities of the SO associated with typical biliary pain. Biliary SO dysfunction must be differentiated from structural diseases such as pancreatitis or a small stone in the bile ducts. Other painful functional disorders such as dyspepsia, IBS, and functional abdominal pain are far more common. The only method that can directly assess the motor function of the SO is manometry—a technique not universally available and with serious complications like pancreatitis. There are three types of functional biliary SO disorder:

- Type I patients have biliary-type pain with (1) transient twice-normal increases in LFTs, (2) increased conjugated bilirubin on two or more occasions, and (3) dilation of the common bile duct to greater than 8mm as determined by ultrasonography.
- Type II patients have biliary pain and fewer than three of the above criteria.
- Type III patients have only recurrent biliary pain.

Functional Pancreatic SO Disorder

This uncommon disorder is characterized by recurrent episodes of epigastric pain that radiates to the back, elevated pancreatic enzymes, and motility abnormalities of the pancreatic SO. Known causes of pancreatitis such as alcohol abuse, gallstones, drugs, or heredity are absent. Attacks are sometimes accompanied by elevated pancreatic enzymes without manifest pancreatitis, but it is uncertain if pancreatic SO dysfunction causes acute pancreatitis.

Tests employed to investigate functional pancreatic SO disorder resemble those of the other functional biliary disorders. The use of ERCP risks pancreatitis, especially if manometry or another bile duct procedure is performed. This uncommon disorder should be managed only where expertise is available. Patients contemplating invasive investigation of the biliary tract and possible remedial endoscopic or surgical correction of the sphincter should be aware of potentially serious complications and treatment failures. An independent second opinion is wise.

Conclusion

This chapter reviews FGIDs that were not discussed in previous chapters. Bloating is a very common, perplexing, and bothersome symptom that is commonly found in IBS and dyspepsia. Nausea and vomiting disorders such as cyclic vomiting can be debilitating, but are fortunately uncommon. Even more troubling is FAPS, which often has major psychological comorbidity. Functional biliary disorders are rarely encountered or recognized and are subject to potentially dangerous investigation. These important symptoms and syndromes challenge researchers to find explanations and more effective treatments.

Sources

Behar J, Corazziari E, Guelrud M, Hogan WJ, Sherman S, Toouli J. Functional gallbladder and sphincter of Oddi disorders. In: Drossman DA, Corazziari E, Delvaux M, Spiller RC, Talley NJ, Thompson WG, Whitehead WE, eds. *Rome III:*

The Functional Gastrointestinal Disorders. McLean, VA: Degnon Associates, Inc; 2006: 595-635.

Clouse RE, Meyer EA, Aziz Q, Drossman DA, Dumitrascu DL, Mönnikes H, Naliboff BD. Functional abdominal pain syndrome. In: Drossman DA, Corazziari E, Delvaux M, Spiller RC, Talley NJ, Thompson WG, Whitehead WE, eds. *Rome III: The Functional Gastrointestinal Disorders.* McLean, VA: Degnon Associates, Inc.; 2006:557-493.

Longstreth GF, Thompson WG, Chey WD, Houghton LA, Mearin F, Spiller RC. Functional bowel disorders. In: Drossman DA, Corazziari E, Delvaux M, Spiller RC, Talley NJ, Thompson WG, Whitehead WE, eds. *Rome III: The Functional Gastrointestinal Disorders.* McLean, VA: Degnon Associates, Inc.; 2006:487-555.

Ringel Y, Drossman DA, Leserman JL, Suyenobu BY, Wilber K, Lin W, Whitehead WE, Naliboff BD, BermanS, Mayer EA. Effect of abuse history on pain reports and brain responses to aversive visceral stimulation: an fMRI study. *Gastroenterology.* 2008;134:396–404

Tack J, Talley NJ, Camilleri M, Holtmann G, Hu P, Malagelada J-R, Stanghellini V. Functional gastroduodenal disorders. In: Drossman DA, Corazziari E, Delvaux M, Spiller RC, Talley NJ, Thompson WG, Whitehead WE, eds. *Rome III: The Functional Gastrointestinal Disorders.* McLean, VA: Degnon Associates, Inc.; 2006:419-485.

PART 3: Managing the Functional Gastrointestinal Disorders

Introduction

In parts 1 and 2 we discussed the nature and diagnosis of the functional gastrointestinal disorders (FGIDs). In part 3, we will address their treatment. Chapter 13 commences with the general treatment measures that are suitable for any of the FGIDs. These include common-sense advice about diagnosis, diet, lifestyle, and the management of stress. A successful therapeutic relationship is essential to achieve the maximum therapeutic benefit. Therefore, this vital interaction is analyzed in chapter 14.

A strong placebo benefit accompanies most FGID treatments, and many symptoms tend to improve naturally. Therefore, it is important that specific treatments should be proven to be of further benefit, and to be safe. This is accomplished through randomized clinical trials (RCTs), which are examined in chapter 15. Such trials are the bedrock of evidence-based medicine. Armed with evidence from RCTs, we can judge which treatments are best for individual patients with FGIDs.

Treatment options that are recommended for specific FGIDs are reviewed in chapter 16. These options constitute a menu from which the treatment most suited to the patient's needs and circumstances can be chosen. To facilitate this choice, the medical evidence supporting them is briefly considered. For many of the treatments, such medical evidence is scant. Some of the more complex of these treatments are discussed in detail in chapter 17.

13 General Treatment Measures

Introduction

The functional gastrointestinal disorders (FGIDs) share distressing, but not life-threatening or disabling symptoms, great prevalence, chronicity, unknown cause(s), and many unproven treatments. Commonly a patient may have more than one disorder. As pointed out in chapter 5, more severely affected patients may also have functional disorders involving body systems other than the gastrointestinal tract. Indeed, it has been claimed that in patients with many somatic symptoms, diagnosis depends upon the specialists to whom they are directed. Henningsen and others use the term *functional somatic syndromes* (table 13-1), and propose a general approach that would embrace many disorders in other body systems as well as the irritable bowel syndrome (and presumably the other functional gastrointestinal disorders). This idea implies a breadth of view that stretches beyond the doctor's immediate specialty and draws attention to the need for a comprehensive and biopsychosocial approach. Some people would argue that in an ideal world a patient with such diverse disorders would best be managed by a general physician—a primary care doctor.

A further shared characteristic, at least in more severely affected patients, is a greater than expected association with psychological problems such as anxiety, depression, and a history of physical or sexual abuse. Few physicians can be expected to be expert in such a wide range of issues, but an approach to them is ventured in this chapter. While a book of functional gut disorders must deal with issues germane to the gut, physicians, patients and other interested people must be mindful of the larger implications. To ignore a patient's other somatic and psychological complaints is both a disservice and a formula for failed management. Physicians who insist on one complaint per visit will be ill-equipped to satisfactorily manage many FGID patients.

The Therapeutic Relationship

The therapeutic relationship is so important to the successful management of the FGIDs that I devote all of chapter 14 to it. However, a few observations

Table 13-1. The Functional Somatic Syndromes*

Irritable bowel syndrome	Chronic pelvic pain
Chronic fatigue syndrome	*Chronic whiplash syndrome*
Fibromyalgia	*Chronic Lyme disease*
Multiple chemical sensitivity	*Silicone breast implant effects*
Nonspecific chest pain	*Candidiasis hypersensitivity*
Premenstrual syndrome	*Mitral valve prolapse*
Repetitive strain injury	*Hypoglycemia*
Tension headache	Chronic low back pain
Temporomandibular joint disorder	Dizziness
Atypical facial pain	*Interstitial cystitis*
Hyperventilation syndrome	Tinnitus
Globus syndrome	Pseudoseizures
Sick building syndrome	Insomnia

Italics indicate conditions whose inclusion here is controversial
Adapted from Henningsen et al, 2007

are appropriate here. The relationship should be established at the first clinical encounter and be maintained throughout all subsequent encounters. Patients should look for doctors who devote sufficient time to understand and deal with their complaints, and who have the patience to provide the empathy and careful explanation that every patient deserves. A successful therapeutic relationship is facilitated if the physician understands why the patient is consulting him. Some of these reasons may not be immediately apparent (see table 13-2).

Medical History

A good medical school curriculum devotes many hours to the very difficult task of interviewing patients and recording an accurate and adequate medi-

Table 13-2. The Reason for the Visit Is Important

Possible Causes That May Prompt an FGID Patient to Consult a Doctor
1. New exacerbating factors (dietary change, concurrent medical disorder, side effects of new medication)
2. Personal concern about a serious disease (recent family death)
3. Environmental stressors (e.g., major loss, abuse history)
4. Psychiatric comorbidity (depression, anxiety)
5. Impairment in daily function (recent inability to work or socialize)
6. A "hidden agenda" such as narcotic or laxative abuse, or pending litigation or disability settlement

Adapted from *Rome III: The Functional Gastrointestinal Disorders*, p. 13.

cal history. This is a complex intellectual and interpersonal exercise that cannot be delegated or accomplished by a questionnaire. The FGIDs will never be properly diagnosed or managed by computer. The medical history should record the chief complaint followed by the details of its occurrence and development. FGID symptoms and red flags should be noted. The doctor should inquire about contributing factors discussed in earlier chapters. She should also know about the patient's prior illnesses and medical procedures, as well as inheritable diseases in parents or siblings, such as colon cancer or inflammatory bowel disease. Relevant life events such as loss of job, bereavement, or other personal tragedy are important, as are prior physical or sexual abuse and psychological illness. As a prelude to recognizing factors that contribute to a patient's distress, a physician should know about his lifestyle, including sexual orientation, diet, tobacco, street drug and alcohol use, and use of prescription drugs.

A doctor must understand what her patient expects or wishes from the consultation. Does he expect a cure, something to relieve the symptoms, or simply reassurance that the condition is benign, and that all the important issues are being addressed? Sometimes, the initial complaint is not the real problem and the patient has another agenda that he is initially reluctant to discuss. These might include a psychological or sexual problem, fear of cancer or other disease, breakdown of a relationship, a difficult family member, or a frustrating job (table 13-2). Superficially, some of these expectations and agendas may seem irrelevant, but frequently they lie at the core of the problem and are the key to managing the patient's investigation and treatment.

Quality of Life (QOL) and Degree of Daily Functioning

Briefly stated, quality of life (QOL) is a person's perception of how well he is able to meet his needs in self-care, physical activities, work, social interactions, and psychological well-being. The health-related quality of life (HRQOL) questionnaire is an instrument meant to measure the impact of a disease or illness on a person's life in terms of personal, marital, and employment happiness, and is proposed as a measure of treatment efficacy. Most HRQOL questionnaires assess daily function or work capability. Some questionnaires are specially designed to measure QOL in patients with FGIDs; the questions they ask are specific to the disorder (e.g., need to be near a bathroom). Disease-specific HRQOL is proposed as a measure of treatment outcome in clinical trials.

The concept of QOL is difficult to apply to the FGIDs, since HRQOL measurements are seldom truly disease-specific. The concept originated as a measure of a person's quality of life in treated and untreated cancer patients; that is, it was a means of determining if the treatment offered an improvement over the disease. One's mind may be focused when diagnosed with cancer; under such circumstances a person may well be capable of comparing QOL off or on treatment for a slow and relentless disease. On the other hand, how one might feel about, respond to, and cope with the chronic, non-life-threatening FGIDs depends upon many things apart from the symptoms themselves. Personality may determine whether a person continues to work and engage socially, despite the symptoms. Somatic symptoms are much more difficult to endure if one is anxious, depressed, or under stress. Fear of serious disease also undermines QOL, as can another person's dismissal that the symptoms are trivial. FGIDs often appear to be precipitated by stressful life events or concurrent somatic symptoms that themselves impact QOL.

Closely related to QOL is how one copes. An individual with an FGID may refuse to give up social or work activities, and carry on despite the symptoms. Another with apparently similar symptoms may be an invalid. A compassionate physician will assess a person's quality of life and determine which factors most likely impair it. Used in this way, an HRQOL assessment is a valuable management tool. It seems a less apt method of measuring response to treatment of an FGID in a clinical trial.

Psychosocial History

Earlier chapters emphasize the association of the FGIDs with various psychosocial states. Previous or existing psychological disorders or physical or sexual abuse are important to know about, as are the patient's use of medications for anxiety, depression, panic or other psychological disturbance. Table 5-2 lists items that help screen for the presence of psychological disorders.

Do FGID symptoms cause absenteeism, sexual and physical dysfunction, impaired relationships, sadness, anger, home confinement, job and marital dissatisfaction? Or is it vice-versa? Do they occur together by coincidence? Or perhaps they are all part of the same process—a biopsychosocial reaction to an environmental stress? What aspects of the FGID most trouble the patient? Whether symptoms come before, after, or coincident with psychosocial distress, the relationship is important. A careful physician will want to understand an FGID patient's psychosocial difficulty before formulating a management plan. The QOL and functionality associated with a functional disorder are unlikely to improve without management of both somatic *and* psychological symptoms.

Diagnostic Testing

One advantage of a prompt provisional diagnosis is that it can focus the investigation. For example, a functional bowel disorder diagnosis would prompt investigation of the intestines, not the stomach or esophagus. Functional diarrhea implies tests for other causes of persistent loose or watery stools, and dyspepsia suggests that ulcers should be excluded by a stomach and duodenum examination. Further afield, fibromyalgia might indicate that joint x-rays are in order, and one might consider a CT scan of the head for someone with headaches. Whatever the diagnosis, the ordered tests should be germane to the body system and anatomical location of the symptom, and should be intended to rule out a competing disease. Unnecessary tests and "diagnostic fishing trips" are costly, waste time, cause adverse effects, and breed patient frustration and anxiety.

Someone undergoing a diagnostic test should know its purpose. He should also understand that a negative test is good news, and have that concept reinforced when the test is complete. Without guidance, a negative test may seem to deepen the mystery. In one study, half the patients seen by their family doctors for IBS feared they had cancer after the encounter, but they were neither told the functional diagnosis, nor reassured. The diagnosis of a functional disorder is made by recognition of the characteristic symptoms, the lack of alarm symptoms, and sometimes normal tests that negate other possible diseases. A thorough, sympathetic review of the pertinent test results and answers to any questions help patients understand their meaning and provide them the reassurance they seek.

Confident Diagnosis

For the functional disorders, a confident and positive diagnosis is essential. It can usually be arrived at in the first interview after a history, physical examination, consideration of the *Rome* criteria, and attention to alarm symptoms. The physician should promptly state the FGID diagnosis if she believes it so. She might suggest that one or two tests be done to exclude an unlikely competing disease, but indicate that she expects them to be negative. With such a briefing, the patient will not be "disappointed" when the test is normal. As part of the diagnosis, the doctor should note any accompanying somatic and psychological disorders. When the tests are complete she may confirm the diagnosis and explain its nature. Only with a confident diagnosis can the patient be reassured and begin to better cope with his symptoms. Brody was an early advocate of the placebo response and the power of reassurance. (See "Sources" at the end of this chapter.) He believes that a diagnosis provides an understandable and satisfying explanation of an illness, indicates that the doctor has taken the symptoms seriously and, now that the problem is known, doctor and patient can begin to seek appropriate treatment. Diagnosis provides meaning for a patient's suffering.

Explanation and Reassurance

A diagnosis should provide meaning and context for the symptoms. FGIDs are very common, and we know how they usually behave. Patients should understand the FGIDs' lack of mortal or physically disabling complications. They should also understand that the symptoms are chronic and/or recurrent. Most people with an FGID will experience the symptoms from time to time throughout their lifetimes. FGIDs do not predispose to serious gastrointestinal disease. There are few specific treatments and a spontaneous and lasting cure is unusual. Although the symptoms seldom permanently go away, there is much that one can do to assuage and cope with them. A positive attitude on the part of the doctor should encourage similar, realistic optimism in the patient.

General measures and diet should be discussed in the light of the specific complaints. Many patients have phobias such as using public toilets, eating out, or the need to ask a hostess for the use of her toilet. These should be discussed and strategies developed to deal with them.

Many patients feel that physicians think their symptoms are "all in their head." Such a notion should be promptly rejected. Many people are not receptive to a psychological diagnosis, even if it is anxiety or depression. Nevertheless, psychological problems are real and, in the context of the FGIDs, must be dealt with along with the equally real somatic symptoms.

If needed, drugs should be offered as palliation rather than cure. Since so many patients consult practitioners of complimentary and alternative medicine, these treatments should be discussed nonjudgmentally. They need not be discouraged, but everyone should appreciate the absence of scientific evidence that they are effective. Patients should be aware that uncertified herbal medicines may be toxic to liver and kidneys, and that contaminated acupuncture needles have transmitted infectious diseases.

Appropriate Treatment

Specific treatments for individual FGIDs are discussed in chapters 16 and 17. There are many, and most of them are of unproven or uncertain efficacy. Even some of those that are evidence-based are only necessary or even practical for more severely affected patients. Within groups of FGID patients exists a spectrum of severity (figure 2-5), which suggests a graded therapeutic response (figure 13-1). Most people with functional gut symptoms do not consult doctors and apparently cope well on their own. Mildly affected patients who are seen in primary care are concerned about the meaning of their symptoms ("Is it cancer?"), and may be satisfied with a diagnosis, prognosis, explanation, and some diet and lifestyle advice. More severely affected patients have continuing symptoms that are often complicated by stress or psychological difficulties that impair QOL. These patients require follow-up visits during which stress management and specific therapies may be tried.

The most severely affected people are a small percentage of all those with FGIDs. They may be deeply distressed, and often their marital, work, and social functioning are impaired. The FGID symptoms, while dominant, may owe their disabling characteristics to the coincident presence of other physical and psychological disturbances. Such patients need specialized care, either in a medical center with medical, psychological, and social services equipped to deal with their complicated problems, or through referral to a mental health

Graded Treatment Response

- Multidisciplinary approach
- Psychological treatments
- Improve functioning

Severe

- Manage stress
- Pharmacotherapy

Moderate

- Diet, lifestyle advice
- Positive diagnosis
- Explain and reassure

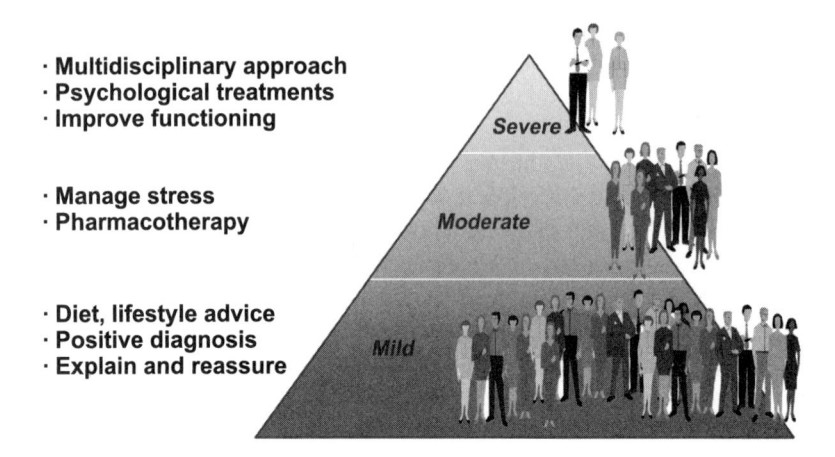

Mild

Figure 13-1. Mildly affected patients in primary care are usually satisfied with a positive diagnosis, explanation, reassurance, and diet and lifestyle advice. The moderately severe may require follow-up visits, referral to a specialist, stress management, and drugs to treat the most troublesome symptoms. Severely affected patients need continuing care, efforts to improve functioning, and possible referral to a mental health professional for psychological or psychopharmaceutical treatments.

professional. In addition, they will require continuing care, either by the medical center or, preferably, by a primary care doctor who is positioned to deal with the patient's community and family relationships.

Patients may move from one category to another, and assessment of current symptom severity can help determine the intensity of treatment. In the absence of cure, an ideal would be to manage the symptoms of FGID patients such that they can cope on their own with a satisfactory QOL. Meanwhile, treatment should be designed to meet an individual patient's needs.

Conclusion

With FGIDs, as with other chronic illnesses, a satisfactory doctor/patient therapeutic relationship is fundamental to successful outcomes. Treatment begins with a thorough medical history that includes family illnesses and co-existing somatic and psychological complaints. The doctor must understand the patient's quality of life, his level of daily functioning, and what perturbs him, including social and psychological difficulties. Diagnostic testing should be brief, directed according to the symptoms, and fully explained before and after any investigation. A confident diagnosis should be made as soon as possible, ideally at the first visit, and serve as platform from which to explain the illness and offer a reassuring, but realistic prognosis. When a diagnosis is made, treatment should be designed on the basis of severity to meet the individual patient's needs.

Sources

Brody H. The placebo response: recent research and implications for family practice. *J Fam Pract.* 2000;47:649-654.

Drossman DA. The functional gastrointestinal disorders and the *Rome III* process. In: Drossman DA, Corazziari E, Delvaux M, Spiller RC, Talley NJ, Thompson WG, Whitehead WE, eds. *Rome III: The Functional Gastrointestinal Disorders.* McLean, VA: Degnon Associates Inc.; 2006:1-30.

Drossman DA, Thompson WG. Irritable bowel syndrome: A graduated, multicomponent treatment approach. *Ann Intern Med.* 1992;116:1009-1016.

Henningsen P, Zipfel S, Herzog W. Management of functional somatic syndromes. *Lancet.* 2007;369(9565):946-955.

Talley NJ. *Conquering Irritable Bowel Syndrome.* Hamilton, ON: B.C.Decker, 2005.

Thomas KB. General practice consultations: is there any point in being positive? *Br Med J.* 1987;294:1200-1202.

Thompson WG, Heaton KW. *Fast Facts: Irritable Bowel Syndrome,* 2nd ed. Oxford: Health Press; 2003.

Thompson WG, Heaton KW, Smyth T, Smyth C. Irritable bowel syndrome in general practice: prevalence, management and referral. *Gut.* 2000;46:78-82.

Wessely S, Mimnuan C, Sharpe M. Functional somatic syndromes: one or many? *Lancet.* 1999;354:936-939.

14 The Therapeutic Relationship: Doctors, Patients, and the Placebo Effect

Introduction
This chapter has two objectives. The first is to demonstrate the powerful healing properties of a good therapeutic relationship between doctor and patient and examine some of the attributes that enhance that relationship. The second is to remind readers that because of the healing attributes of the therapeutic relationship, treatment should as far as possible be guided by scientific evidence. To provide necessary background for these objectives, I will first review two important and germane concepts: the natural history of chronic diseases such as the functional gastrointestinal disorders (FGIDs) and the placebo effect. By augmenting the intrinsic benefit of a treatment, time and placebo effects become indispensable components of therapeutic success. Their exploitation depends upon a satisfactory doctor/patient relationship.

Components of a Therapeutic Response
Figure 14-1 illustrates a hypothetical twelve-week clinical trial of a chronic, painful condition such as irritable bowel syndrome, dyspepsia, or fibromyalgia. Two groups of similar patients are randomly allocated to receive either a new drug being tested for the disorder or an identically appearing inert pill—a placebo. The symptoms are assessed weekly by a global outcome measure that embraces pain and well-being. The weekly assessments continue over a four-week follow-up period. This is an example of a randomized clinical trial (RCT). (RCTs are discussed in more detail in the next chapter.)

In figure 14-1, the patients whose conditions improved on the test drug are indicated in black and those on placebo in grey. About 50% and 40% of the patients in their respective groups are improved. The difference between the two sets of values, about 10%, is known as the *therapeutic gain*. In this case, let us assume it achieves statistical significance—that is, the test drug is deemed to be more effective than placebo. However, in this chapter we are interested in what is happening to the patients in the placebo group, for after all, 40%

Components of a Therapeutic Outcome

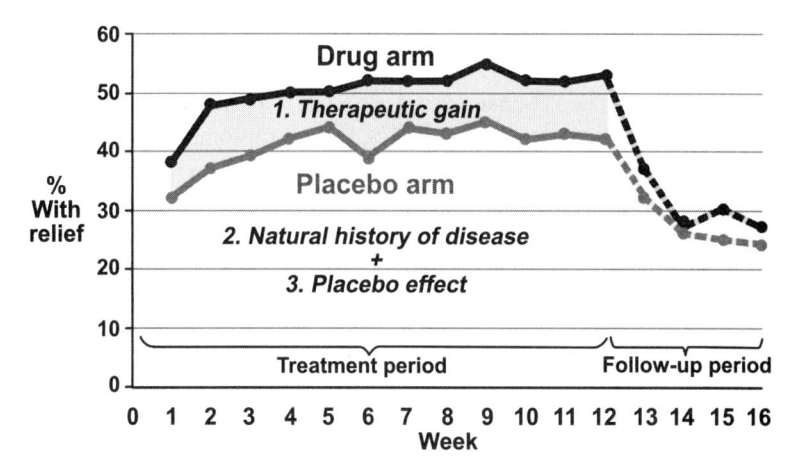

Figure 14-1. A hypothetical, twelve-week randomized clinical trial and four-week follow-up for a chronic, painful disorder where the global outcome measure was "relief of pain and restored well-being." The diagram illustrates three components of a therapeutic benefit. The difference between the number of improved patients in the drug and placebo groups (shaded area) is the *therapeutic gain*—during the twelve-week treatment period, the drug relieves the pain 'significantly' better than placebo. The gain of about 10% seems superficially disappointing, but is similar to the therapeutic gains of many drugs approved by regulatory authorities. About 40% of the patients in the placebo group are improved. When the drug and placebo are discontinued, the number of responders drops dramatically to the same level, about 25%. The drop to 25% may represent the loss of the placebo effect in both groups of patients plus the loss of the therapeutic gain in the drug-treated patients. The natural history of painful conditions is for the pain to fluctuate in intensity. Therefore, the approximate 25% improvement over baseline after follow-up may indicate where the improved subjects would have been had no treatment been given. (See the text for caveats.) Placebo effects and natural improvement are at work in every successful therapeutic encounter. In FGIDs, they may be the most powerful determinants of a treatment's success. (Adapted from Thompson WG, 2005.)

of them are improved with no specific treatment. As indicated in the figure, there are two main components to this improvement: the natural history of the disease and the placebo effect.

Natural History of the Disease

The FGIDs are chronic, relapsing disorders; their symptoms wax and wane. If the symptoms are waxing at the time of entry into the trial (as they would be to justify treatment), many patients would be expected to improve over the sixteen weeks of the trial and follow-up. Thus, in the placebo group, many patients would naturally improve even if a trial had not taken place. However, a trial such as the one illustrated in figure 12-1 is not a natural history experiment. Any treatment is an intervention that may influence outcome. Examples include parallel interventions for all study participants, such as diet and medication adjustment, and ready access to advice from trial doctors and nurses. Nevertheless, as healers have known since tribal days, many symptoms improve simply with the passage of time.

The Placebo Effect

The placebo effect is demonstrated in figures 14-2a and 14-2b. A general practitioner in England gathered two hundred consecutive patients in four groups of fifty each. All had complaints for which no diagnosis was attached, many of which probably constituted functional somatic disorders such as the FGIDs. In the figure, the two groups above the dashed line received a diagnosis by the doctor and were told that they would improve. The patients in the second of those groups also received inert pills and were told the pills would help. The two groups below the dashed line received no diagnosis and were told that the doctor did not know what they had. The patients in the second of those groups were also given pills, but the doctor told them that he did not know if they would help. At a subsequent visit (figure 14-2b), 64% of the patients were improved in the two groups above the dashed line, and only 39% in the groups below the line.

In other words, through a diagnosis and a positive attitude on the part of the doctor, 25% more patients improved than otherwise would have done so. The giving or not giving of pills made no difference to the outcome. An inert pill, sham operation, or blinded procedure might have no influence on the outcome of an illness, but the positive attitude of the doctor who "cares" to give a diagnosis can have a powerful effect. It is the placebo *effect* that is important, not the placebo—and the doctor is the key.

The Therapeutic Equation

Now let us look again at the trial depicted in figure 14-1. It is incorrect to assume that the apparent drug benefit of 50% is entirely due to the properties of the drug. Indeed, if the trial is properly designed and blinded, then what is

Figure 14-2. The importance of a diagnosis and a positive attitude and the irrelevance of pills.

The Power of a Positive Message
in 200 GP patients with indefinite diagnosis

N	Diagnosis	Doctor attitude
50	Yes	"You will be better soon."
50	Yes + pills	"Pills will help."
50	No	"I don't know what . . ."
50	No + pills	"I don't know if . . ."

A. Two hundred consecutive general practice (GP) patients with uncertain diagnoses were divided into two groups randomly. The patients in the first two groups (above the dotted line) were given diagnoses and told they would get better. The second of these first two groups were given pills and told the pills would help. The other two groups (below the dashed line) were given no diagnosis and were told that the doctor did not know what they had. Patients in the second of these two groups received pills but were told that the doctor was uncertain if they would help.

The Power of a Positive Message
in 200 GP patients with indefinite diagnosis

Improved
$P<.001$

Diagnosis & positive	32/50	
Diagnosis & positive + pill	32/50	64%
No diagnosis	18/50	
No diagnosis + pill	21/50	39%

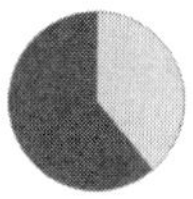

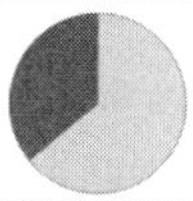

B. At follow-up, 64% of the patients who received a diagnosis and positive attitude (above the dashed line) were improved, while only 39% of those who received no diagnosis and a neutral approach were better. Whether pills were given did not affect the outcome.

120 Understanding the Irritable Gut

Figure 14-3. Recreation of the hypothetical trial from figure 14-1, where the placebo and time effects are removed from the treatment results. Assuming this were possible, the improvement would be then entirely due to the therapeutic gain, a mere 10%.

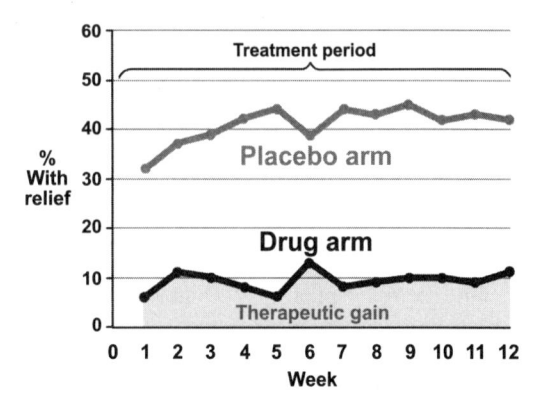

happening to the group on placebo is exactly duplicated in the drug-treated group except for the test drug's effect. When one strips away the natural history and placebo benefits, the drug's advantage is confined to its therapeutic gain, which at 10% seems hardly worth prescribing (figure 14-3). These therapeutic components in a group of treated subjects can be expressed in the following way:

Therapeutic benefit = therapeutic gain + natural history + placebo effect

Wise healers know this instinctively and attempt to bring all three components to bear when treating an illness. Readers will now recognize that all three need not be positive to achieve a benefit. In an *uncontrolled* clinical trial, a powerful placebo effect and a favorable natural history may make a useless treatment appear effective. In other words, the power of the physician-patient interaction can make treatments successful. Thus,

Therapeutic benefit = no therapeutic gain + natural history + placebo effect

Clinical trials were invented in the 1930s and 1940s, which means that evidence-based medicine is little more than half a century old. Before that time conventional doctors employed many useless treatments with little proof that they were effective. For centuries dangerous treatments such as venesection (blood letting), purging, and lengthy bed rest for a wide range of ailments killed more people than they cured. Hence,

Therapeutic benefit = therapeutic loss + natural history + placebo effect

Such placebo and time effects mask the therapeutic inutility—and even the harm—of many contemporary FGID treatments. Clinical trial results provide the data we must rely upon to avoid such clinical misinformation. Unfortunately, evidence-based medicine has limits. There are far too few resources and investigator personnel to test every proposed treatment. For some treatments such as psychotherapy it is difficult to design suitable controls. Surgical placebos are rarely possible for obvious ethical and practical reasons. Withholding therapy in placebo-control groups is sometimes problematic. Individualized treatments such as diet, homeopathy, and hypnosis do not easily lend themselves to randomization. Nevertheless, the RCT is the best tool we have to ensure that an FGID treatment is rational, effective, and safe. Surely, any proposed new treatment must be so evaluated.

The Nocebo Effect

If a physician's positive attitude and diagnosis can improve treatment outcomes, a perceived negative attitude and no diagnosis—that is, an unsatisfactory therapeutic relationship—may have a *nocebo* effect that compromises the outcome. Breakdown in the therapeutic relationship can result from a doctor's hurried, uncaring manner, miscommunication, and a host of other negative human interactions. These have the potential for great harm. In this case, the following equation applies:

Therapeutic harm = therapeutic gain + natural history - nocebo effect

Note that a strong nocebo effect may overwhelm any therapeutic gain.

The Therapeutic Relationship

The importance of a good therapeutic relationship in diagnosing and managing the FGIDs is emphasized throughout the *Rome III* book. Guidelines are proposed that may help physicians to establish such a relationship (table 14-1). Most of these are practical, common-sense principles that facilitate a diagnostic conclusion and permit one to develop a management plan. However, inherent in each guideline are opportunities for doctors and patients to establish a human relationship. By following these guidelines a physician communicates compassion and concern for the patient's problems. The patient may sense that someone is now taking care of him. Moreover, if the relationship is successful, he is more likely to adhere to a treatment program.

Respect for the patient is implicit in each of the guidelines. Items 5, 8, and 9 provide opportunities for patients to share responsibility for their care. Guideline 10 acknowledges the multifaceted issues that confront the patient. A primary care physician knows the community where the patient lives and likely knows the family as well. Such knowledge and the community doctor's breadth of experience can help her deal with problems outside a specialist's purview. Liaison between specialists and other health and mental health care personnel who treat functional somatic syndromes is important and best orchestrated by a general physician.

Table 14-1. Guidelines for the Establishment of a Therapeutic Relationship

1. Obtain the history through a nondirective, nonjudgmental, patient-centered interview.
2. Conduct a careful examination and cost-efficient investigation.
3. Determine the patient's understanding of the illness and his or her concerns. *("What do you think is causing your symptoms?")*
4. Provide a thorough explanation of the disorder that takes into consideration the patient's beliefs.
5. Identify and respond realistically to the patient's expectations for improvement. *("How do you feel I can be helpful to you?")*
6. When possible, provide a link between stressors and symptoms that are consistent with patient's beliefs. *("I understand you don't think stress is causing your pain, but the pain itself is so severe and disabling that it's causing you a great deal of distress.")*
7. Set consistent limits. *("I appreciate how bad the pain must be, but narcotic medication is not indicated.")*
8. Involve the patient in the treatment. *("Let me suggest some treatments for you to consider.")*
9. Make recommendations consistent with patient interests. *("Antidepressants can be used for depression, but they are also used to 'turn down' the pain, and in doses lower than those used for depression.")*
10. Establish a long-term relationship with a primary care provider.

Adapted from *Rome III: The Functional Gastrointestinal Disorders*, pp. 12-13.

How the Therapeutic Relationship Works

In this age of medical technology, the belief is common that medicine is a commodity that can be purchased as a unit. Have an infection? Take a pill. Got gall stones? Have them out. If that were true, computers could replace doctors and treatment could be an automatic response to a complaint. Some politicians, managers, and even doctors seem to think that is the case, which leads them to allow health care statistics and demand for procedures to determine policy. The truth is much more nuanced. Most medical encounters require no technology. Indeed every patient needs the careful assessment described in chapter 5. Performing such an assessment is a challenging interpersonal skill that can neither be computerized nor delegated. Moreover, the foregoing discussion of the healing benefit of time and the placebo response should convince us that there is much more to healing than eliminating disease.

Disease is usually accompanied by illness—the pain, disability, suffering, and ominous meaning attached to the symptoms. Even when a person is suffering a terminal disease, his illness can be alleviated by compassion and by careful and collaborative deployment of the available treatment options. In

14. The Therapeutic Relationship: Doctors, Patients, and the Placebo Effect

the FGIDs, there is no demonstrable disease, but often much illness. Discomfort, embarrassment, fear, and a host of emotions aggravate the symptoms and impair a person's quality of life and functioning. Figures 14-2a and 14-2b illustrate that patients can be improved after clinical encounters with doctors and nurses without any specific treatment. There are no objective measures here—no shrunken cancers or decreased fever—but only the extent to which the patient feels better. This can best be achieved by wise exploitation of the placebo effect and of the tendency of most symptoms in most people to improve with time. That these effects are difficult to measure is granted, but they are nonetheless important. Regrettably, they seem not to influence health care policy.

If the placebo effect is so important, we should examine what optimizes it. Because it occurs through the therapeutic or doctor/patient relationship, we should begin there. Some improvement can be attributed to conditioning. If previous visits have had good outcomes, the patient may be conditioned to respond likewise this time. If a placebo is given *after* a course of an effective drug, it will be more effective than if it were given first.

Expectation and desire are important as well. Because a patient believes that a doctor or other healer will help him, then she is more likely to do so. In one experiment, a pain-causing substance was injected into the skin of all four limbs of volunteers. Randomly, an inert cream was applied to some of the limbs, where it relieved the pain. The volunteers expected the cream to relieve the pain in the treated limbs, and it did. If you believe a substance such as caffeine or alcohol will somehow improve your performance, it is more likely to do so than if you have doubts. A patient's expectations of the doctor/healer and their perceived realization during the consultation can reinforce the benefits of treatment.

It is said that the doctor *is* the placebo. How is this so? There appear to be many factors at work. The doctor's reputation, profession, and demeanor build confidence. As figure 14-2 illustrates, the confidence, enthusiasm, and positivity with which a doctor delivers care can enhance the benefit. Even the office or clinic can create an atmosphere of healing with its medicinal smells, diplomas, instruments, and bustling activity. The examination itself, sometimes dismissively called the "laying on of hands," can be comforting. "At last, someone is taking my problem seriously!"

Figure 14-2 also illustrates the importance of a diagnosis in providing meaning for a patient. Only after diagnosis can the doctor and patient take the opportunity to discuss such things as prognosis, risks, and the nature of the illness. Only at that point can the doctor provide the reassurance most patients with functional somatic complaints need, particularly if they have come to the doctor because they were in fear of serious disease.

The three dimensions of a symptom such as pain were introduced in chapter twelve (figure 12-1). The *sensory-discrimination dimension* occurs typically when one is injured, such as when inadvertently striking one's thumb with a hammer. Nerve endings in the thumb instantly send messages to the brain, and we feel pain. A disease equivalent might be acute appendicitis, where the appendix's nerve endings rapidly transmit pain signals to the brain. In either case, some relief can be achieved with analgesics (pain killers). The *affective-motivational dimension* is most prominent in chronic pain, such as in some FGIDs, where description and location of the pain are indistinct. Anxiety is commonly present. *The cognitive-behavioral dimension* generates fear, worry, and frustration. In chronic pain, wherein the patient has more time to contemplate the symptom, the latter two dimensions obscure the sensory-discriminatory dimension. Analgesic drugs are typically ineffective in chronic pain because of these attributes. Relief depends more on the physician's skill in alleviating the anxiety, fear, and worry than on any specific treatment. These affective and cognitive aspects of a chronic, painful illness may require the psychological or psychopharmaceutical approaches that are discussed in chapter 16.

When relief depends heavily upon the physician's skill in alleviating the anxiety, fear, and worry, the physician or healer becomes a healing instrument. She or he can inspire confidence, make a diagnosis, relieve anxiety, assuage fear, and express empathy. This requires time—a commodity not often mentioned in health care debates. The *Rome III* guidelines in table 14-1 cannot be satisfied in a five-minute visit. Since time costs money and both are controlled by third parties, doctors and patients can do little to extend it. Yet sufficient time is so important to the doctor-patient relationship that its provision should be just as much a part of the health care effort as shorter wait times and technological availability. Lack of sufficient time for the therapeutic relationship is a nocebo.

Evidence-based Medicine

The second objective of this chapter is to emphasize that treatment should be guided by medical evidence whenever possible. Ideally, every treatment should be proven to be effective, rather than exclusively exploit the benefits of time and the placebo effect. More importantly, harmful treatments should not be disguised by these effects. Anecdote, clinical experience—even a convincing pathophysiological theory—are insufficient. The evidence must be gathered through randomized, controlled clinical trials (RCTs).

If only it were that simple! There are too many treatments extant—information, diet, exercise, drugs, surgery, alternative medicine, even psychotherapy—to test them all with RCTs. Trials are expensive. They are very difficult to conduct in a truly random population to ensure that they will apply to individuals. Some trials are impossible, such as those for surgery where sham operations would be unacceptable, for psychotherapy where expectations of the test treatment are difficult to control, or for herbal treatments where ingredients vary with the herbal crop and their myriad combinations. If there are no relevant RCTs, clinical judgment must be invoked—provided certain characteristics are observed. Is the treatment plausible? Is the cause of the condition sufficiently understood so that logical countermeasures can be employed? Does the treatment have potential for harm? Does the cost justify the potential benefit? Is it ethical and does the doctor believe it is useful? Does the doctor have any conflict of interest that might bias her clinical judgment?

Despite the foregoing caveats, evidence gathered from RCTs provides important treatment signposts. Frequently, certain practices are proven effective and become widespread as a result of successful trials, and long-lasting traditional treatments are summarily discarded when an RCT fails to demonstrate safety and efficacy. Such trials are the only way that a new treatment can be proven acceptably safe and effective. In the FGIDs, medical evidence is scarce. The development of the *Rome* criteria now permits recognizable patients to be entered in trials and the results to be applied to similar patients in the clinic. Before discussing more specific treatments of the FGIDs, the next chapter will review the elements of an FGID clinical trial.

Conclusion

The placebo effect and the wise exploitation of time's propensity to heal are very important ingredients of the therapeutic relationship and are particularly important in the FGIDs. Their failure can negate the benefit of normally effective therapy. Thus the doctor/patient therapeutic relationship is the most important component of FGID therapy. Conversely, these effects can mask the inutility of a treatment, or even permit the continued use of a harmful one. This forces us to critically appraise all treatments. Although most treatments are not evidence-based, the physician's knowledge of medicine, the patient's personal history, and the accumulated medical evidence should help guide them both to the most effective and safest treatments available. Meanwhile, it is desirable and ethical that healers augment the benefits of legitimate treatments by exploiting the placebo response through an optimum therapeutic relationship.

Sources

Drossman DA. The functional gastrointestinal disorders and the *Rome III* process. In: Drossman DA, Corazziari E, Delvaux M, Spiller RC, Talley NJ, Thompson WG, Whitehead WE, eds. *Rome III: The Functional Gastrointestinal Disorders*. McLean, VA: Degnon Associates, Inc.; 2006:1-30.

Irvine EJ, Whitehead WE, Chey WD, Matsueda K, Shaw M, Talley NJ, van Zanten SV. Design of treatment trials for functional gastrointestinal disorders. In: Drossman DA, Corazziari E, Delvaux M, Spiller RC, Talley NJ, Thompson

WG, Whitehead WE, eds. *Rome III: The Functional Gastrointestinal Disorders.* McLean, VA: Degnon Associates, Inc.; 2006:779-833.

Longstreth GF, Thompson WG, Chey WD, Houghton LA, Mearin F, Spiller RC. The functional bowel disorders. In: Drossman DA, Corazziari E, Delvaux M, Spiller RC, Talley NJ, Thompson WG, Whitehead WE, eds. *Rome III: The Functional Gastrointestinal Disorders.* McLean, VA: Degnon Associates, Inc.; 2006:487-555.

Thomas KB. General practice consultations: is there any point in being positive? *Br Med J.* 1987;294:1200-1202.

Thompson WG. The Placebo Effect in Health: *Combining Science and Compassionate Care.* Amherst, NY: Prometheus, 2005.

15 Proving Treatments Work: Randomized Clinical Trials

> "... while the individual man is an insoluble puzzle, in the aggregate he becomes a mathematical certainty. You can, for example, never foretell what any man will do, but you can say with precision what an average number will be up to. Individuals vary, but percentages remain constant. So says the statistician."
> —Sherlock Holmes in The Sign of the Four, Arthur Conan Doyle

Introduction

A clinical trial is an experiment designed to determine the value of a treatment, prevention measure, or test. It normally requires the participation of representative people or patients at a similar stage of illness or health. When the intervention is compared to another treatment, a placebo, or a sham procedure, and the patients are randomly allocated into treatment and control groups, the experiment is called a *randomized clinical trial* (RCT). The accumulated scientific data from such trials permit the practice of evidence-based medicine.

The Need for Clinical Trials

Some treatments induce a benefit so obvious and dramatic they require no clinical trial to justify them. Examples include insulin for diabetes and penicillin for pneumococcal pneumonia. The advantages of setting a fracture or removing a foreign body are unassailable. However, the efficacy of most treatments and tests is uncertain, particularly for chronic, painful conditions such as the functional gastrointestinal disorders (FGIDs). Some people improve after a treatment, some remain the same, and some worsen. Anecdotal evidence, such as a patient's or a doctor's favorable therapeutic experience, is insufficient justification for its use for others. As implied by Mr. Holmes, only a collective experience can establish whether in similar circumstances a treatment will benefit more people than "no treatment" will.

Some treatments whose utility seems self-evident may be subject to bias. Even if a medicine's potentially useful pharmacological effects provide a scientific rationale, a single happy result is insufficient medical evidence of its usefulness. A doctor administering a treatment believes it will improve symptoms and convinces the patient. If the outcome is good, both are content—but perhaps both are deceived! Because of the placebo effect and the tendency of most illness to improve, the treatment falsely can appear effective. Hence, many treatments appear to "cure" a cold because normally it is over in a week.

If you feel better after a treatment, why question it? Apart from the personal and public deception implied by such an attitude, there are practical reasons for skepticism. Some treatments are costly, and most drugs have adverse effects that offend Hippocrates' ancient admonishment to "do no harm." A drug, operation, diet, or test that harms even one patient is justified only if the disease is sufficiently serious and many other patients can expect to benefit. Ineffective treatments generate false hope and distract from better options.

When improvement of a single patient is unconvincing, therapists may cite a series of patients. A surgeon may claim that a specific operation cures most of his cases. Physicians may adopt a drug that helped someone in the past. All are subject to bias. A treatment's early success through happenstance reinforces its power or credibility, and physicians spread the word to colleagues. Such reinforcement enhances the placebo effect and perpetuates useless treatments. Little is lost if the treatments are inexpensive, harmless, and for minor illness, but greatly publicized and ultimately worthless cancer cures such as Laetrile, or dangerous cure-alls such as venesection (blood-letting), do more harm than good. In an ideal world, all treatments and tests should be scientifically evaluated by RCTs.

Randomized, controlled clinical trials revolutionized how physicians think and practice and RCTs enhance doctors' ability to cure disease and relieve suffering. Regulatory authorities such as the U.S. Food and Drug Administration and the European Agency for the Evaluation of Medicinal Products must approve new drugs before physicians may prescribe them. The approval process requires long, arduous, and expensive RCTs. The failure of new products to be released in a timely manner frustrates many, but the alternative is the ignorant use of costly, useless, and potentially harmful drugs.

Regrettably, few treatments other than new prescription drugs are subject to regulatory scrutiny. Many products were approved long ago, when plausibility and safety were the principle requirements. Now national and managed health care organizations, who must pay the bills, demand medical evidence before placing a drug on their formularies. The marketplace may fill the regulatory void.

Bias

Bias means to influence, sway, or favor an argument. In science, it describes any factor or process that deviates the results or conclusions of an experiment away from the truth. Anecdotes invite bias. When a treatment and a successful outcome occur together, cause and effect may be wrongly assumed. Coincidence does not imply cause. Most illnesses improve with time, and the healer's enthusiasm and the patient's expectations have benefits. How else can one explain the centuries-long use of blood-letting, leeches, ritual purging, and many alternative therapies?

Only by comparison with suitable and contemporaneous controls can a treatment's usefulness be judged. Historical controls, where previous patient outcomes are compared with those after a new treatment, introduce bias if the circumstances change. The enthusiasm of doctors and the hopeful expectations of patients for the new treatment were usually missing during the historical control period. A properly-conducted RCT seeks to avoid such biases. Nevertheless, bias may sully an RCT at any stage from patient selection to analysis (see table 15-1).

Elements of the Ideal Randomized, Controlled Clinical Trial For FGIDs

This section outlines the elements of an ideal RCT for an FGID as conceptualized in *Rome III: The Functional Gastrointestinal Disorders*. Studies of pathophysiology or diagnostic tests require different trial designs and are not

Table 15-1. Major Sources of Bias in RCTs

Bias Type	Comments
1. Investigator bias	Conscious or unconscious bias, often in patient selection
2. Ascertainment bias:	
a. Self-selection for treatment	Patients are more likely to respond positively to treatments they prefer or seek out.
b. Changes in subject pool	Publicity or other factors influence participation.
3. Patient expectancy (placebo)	Especially relevant in unblinded or outcome-subjective trials
4. Nonspecific effects:	
a. Doctor-patient relationship	Important in all interventions, but variable
b. "Regression to the mean"	Subjects who are enrolled when they are most symptomatic inevitably improve.
5. Publication bias	Authors are more likely to submit positive results and medical journals are more likely to publish them.

Adapted from *Rome III: The Functional Gastrointestinal Disorders*, p. 786.

included here. Nevertheless, the scientific principles are similar for all RCTs, and must be understood if physicians and patients are to apply medical evidence when treating FGIDs.

Hypotheses and Outcomes

Treatment trials seek to ascertain the impact of a treatment on the frequency and severity of symptoms, health status, quality of life, or the use of health care resources. To determine one of these outcomes, all other elements of the participants' experience must be held constant; that is, only the test treatment distinguishes treated patients from the controls. A single hypothesis should be stated and a suitable RCT should be designed to prove it or not.

It is best that only one *primary outcome measure* determines the result of the trial. More than one outcome measure weakens the study unless statistical allowance is made—the more questions asked, the more likely a positive answer by chance alone. Of course, subsidiary questions are permissible, but should serve to either support the primary outcome or to generate hypotheses for future testing. For example, in an antidiarrheal drug trial, a primary outcome of improved stool consistency is supported by a secondary outcome of reduced stool frequency. Another secondary outcome, such as improved nutrition, if positive might generate a new hypothesis to be tested by another RCT. Because secondary outcomes are not part of the original hypothesis where statistics properly may be applied, they are weak medical evidence.

Patient Selection and Characteristics

The *Rome* diagnostic criteria made modern FGID trials possible. Without specific biomarkers for the FGIDs, patients can only be identified by their symptoms. Previously, a patient's entry into a trial was based upon a doctor's opinion of the diagnosis or the lack of structural disease. Now, patient-described symptoms determine eligibility. Ideally, trial subjects should include patients whose demographic characteristics and disease state resemble those of patients whom a practicing doctor will likely encounter. An RCT's inclusion and exclusion criteria must be clear. A laxative may be tested on constipated patients, but those with kidney failure might be excluded because they risk electrolyte loss. The resulting data would not be strictly applicable to constipated kidney patients. Similarly, a drug that is proven effective for women with irritable bowel syndrome (IBS) is not necessarily useful in men.

In an FGID trial, a minimum evaluation should include a blood count, recent images of the relevant part of the gastrointestinal tract, and other investigations necessitated by the symptoms and family history. Procedures should be consistent across all study groups. Misdiagnosed patients in a clinical trial confound the results, and missing entry data hamper the analysis.

Trial reports should describe how subjects are recruited. Most FGID trials are conducted in academic centers, which risks a selection bias because their patients have more severe symptoms and psychosocial comorbidity. Evidence from such studies may be inappropriate for primary care patients and irrelevant to those not seeking care. Patients recruited by newspaper advertisements have different demographic and psychological characteristics than those enrolled by physicians.

Patient characteristics may alter an RCT's outcome. These include age, race, symptom severity and duration, prior treatments, and the use of medications such as over-the-counter drugs. There should be sufficient men and women with such characteristics in each treatment group to ensure homogeneity and permit meaningful comparisons.

Blinding, Randomization, and Control Treatments

Treatment trials for the FGIDs are complicated by the placebo response and by fluctuating symptoms. Parallel treatments or drugs taken for other conditions may alter outcomes, and side effects may disclose the treatment. These characteristics make it both essential and difficult to blind patients and investigators.

To eliminate bias, patients and researchers should be ignorant of the allocation of test treatment and control subjects—a process known as *double blinding*. Triple blinding includes all investigators, data managers, and statisticians. To test the blinding, investigators should ask all participants which treatment they believe was administered. Certain treatments are difficult to conceal, such as psychotherapy, hypnosis, or drugs with predictable side effects or rapid symptom change. In such cases, independent assessors, standardized interviews, and self-administered questionnaires help minimize bias.

Randomization is the process, analogous to the flip of a coin, of assigning patients to treatment and control arms of an RCT. Random allocation and blinding ensure that research personnel are unaware of each subject's treatment until after the outcome is determined. A placebo control group is usually essential to establish the efficacy of a new treatment. However, if another treatment has been proven efficacious, it may serve as the control. In psychological treatment trials, it is difficult to mount control treatments that generate expectancy comparable to the test treatment. Untreated patients are poor controls because of their low expectations.

A placebo is an intervention, believed to lack any specific therapeutic effect, that serves as a comparison for the active treatment in a clinical trial. The *placebo effect* is the difference in outcome between a placebo-treated group and an untreated group in an unbiased experiment. (This is a philosophical contradiction—can lack of effect have an effect? But then, there is no flawless definition of the placebo effect.) A placebo administered by a physician appears to be more powerful than one given by other health professionals. A generation ago, doctors deliberately prescribed inert pills as placebo treatments—today a forgotten, empty, and unethical gesture.

Placebo responses of up to 80% occur in FGID trials. Some comparisons demonstrate an "order effect." In crossover trials, approximately half the patients will receive placebo first, which can reduce the subsequent response to the trial treatment. Conversely, a placebo has a greater benefit when given after an effective drug. In attempts to minimize placebo responses, older studies employed a run-in period in which all patients received placebo for a specified period. If an individual significantly improved on the placebo, that person was excluded from further participation so as to eliminate placebo responders. This is mistaken because it fails to change the placebo response rate, exaggerates order effects, and impairs the generalizability of the trial's results. Moreover, if 80% of people feel better with the passage of time and placebo effects, surely a treatment must offer something more!

Trial Design and Conduct of an RCT

Clinical trials differ from clinical practice in several ways: strict eligibility criteria, use of a control group, standardized intervention, extensive data gathering, and frequent visits with study coordinators. Moreover, explanation and reassurance about the disease and the general treatment measures are provided to all trial subjects. Such conditions create a healing environment that encourages a placebo effect. To convince us of their efficacy, novel interventions must demonstrate an improvement over such measures.

A *parallel group study design* requires that, after baseline assessment, patients be randomized to receive one of two treatment assignments. General management must be similar in each treatment group throughout the trial. In some variants of the parallel design more than one control or treatment group may be included, or different groups may receive different doses of the test drug (dose-ranging studies).

In a *crossover design,* subjects successively receive both treatments during distinct periods, separated by a drug "washout" phase. Less variability within the subject population could require fewer participants, but dropout rates and missing data have a greater impact in crossover studies than they do in a parallel design. In addition, order effects (the first treatment influences the response to the second), fluctuating symptoms, and the risk of unblinding due to side effects can obscure the benefits. Crossover designs work best in physiological studies where outcomes are objectively measured.

A *superiority* or *noninferiority* trial is appropriate if an effective treatment is available as a control and, as is the case with cancer, it would be unethical to administer a placebo. Equivalence trials require more subjects because statistically it is more difficult to demonstrate equivalence than a difference between treatments. It is unethical to bias a trial deliberately by comparing a test treatment to an inadequate dose of the comparison treatment.

A trial's duration depends upon the frequency and duration of symptoms. For IBS, flares and remissions appear to last less than a week. Trials of eight to twelve weeks are considered long enough to address the chronic nature of the illness, but lengthy studies are hampered by cost and the ability to retain patients. Now, short-term efficacy trials are usually four weeks, and long-term maintenance trials require at least six months. Acute trials normally include patients who have symptoms at the time of randomization, but long-term studies could include both symptomatic and asymptomatic patients. Extended follow-up is essential to determine the durability and safety of a treatment.

Participants' adherence to or compliance with the treatment protocol can greatly influence trial results. Adherence or lack of it is determined through interviews, unused medication counts, or blood drug levels. Compliant or not, all subjects must be included in an *intention-to-treat* analysis.

Assessing the Outcome

Retrospective questionnaires tend to elicit favorable responses, especially if they are completed in the presence of the investigator. Recall of health-related events appears to be accurate only up to three months. Therefore, patients should complete questionnaires before treatment, at follow-up visits, and at the endpoint. Diaries can measure outcomes and minimize recall bias if they are up-to-date. Electronic means such as hand-held devices with reminder alarms, secure Web sites, or telephone reminders can improve adherence. The primary outcome variable determines the success or failure of a treatment. For reasons stated above, one or at most two primary outcomes should be selected before the trial begins. Secondary outcome results strengthen the primary results if they agree. They may help explain the mechanism of the intervention, assess its safety or cost-effectiveness, and identify those patients most likely to benefit from the intervention.

The common scales that are used to assess symptom severity are *categorical scales* (ordinal or Likert), *visual analogue scales* (VAS) (figure 15-1), and numerical rating scales. A categorical scale has several response categories, each with a verbal descriptor. An odd number of response options permits subjects to select a neutral value. Statistical analysis of differences among responses is possible if the scale intervals are equal. A combined categorical scale is illustrated in table 15-2. "Satisfactory relief" exemplifies a *binary scale* ("yes" vs. "no"). The chosen scale should detect any improvement or deterioration.

Before a trial, investigators must define what constitutes a responder—that is, what measures will identify a subject as someone who has responded to the intervention. The definition should reflect a clinically meaningful symptom improvement for each patient. Unfortunately, for FGIDs there is no consensus

VAS Scale

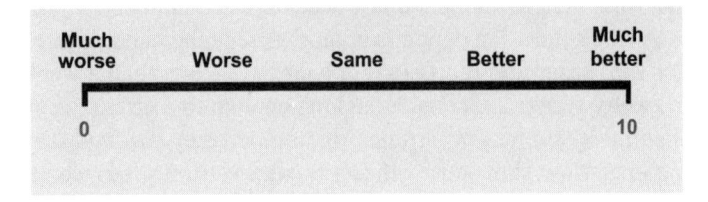

```
Much                                              Much
worse      Worse      Same      Better           better
├─────────────────────────────────────────────────┤
0                                                  10
```

Figure 15-1. Visual Analogue Scale (VAS). Note the balanced scale. A subject marks the horizontal line according to the severity of his symptom (e.g., pain). If this is done before and after the treatment period of a clinical trial, the change in severity is the distance between the two marks. Sufficient improvement can be defined beforehand and used as an outcome measure. (From Thompson WG, 2005, p. 99.)

Table 15-2. Examples of Scales for Measuring RCT Outcome

- Seven-point *Likert scale* for global rating. Patients indicate their improvement from among the following:
  No improvement at all
  Minor improvement
  Mild improvement
  Moderate improvement
  Quite a bit of improvement
  A lot of improvement
  Great improvement

- Combined Scale. Patients first report if they have improved, remained the same, or deteriorated.
  1. Worse
  2. About the same
  3. Better

  If a change occurs, the degree of change is then scored on a seven-point Likert scale, providing a fifteen-point scale of change from –7 to 0 to +7. (Only deterioration is shown below.)
  1. Almost the same, hardly any worse at all
  2. A little worse
  3. Somewhat worse
  4. Moderately worse
  5. A good deal worse
  6. A great deal worse
  7. A very great deal worse

Adapted from *Rome III: The Functional Gastrointestinal Disorders*, p. 810.

on what constitutes a clinically meaningful improvement. Should it be a 10% reduction as rated on a VAS, one step on a seven-step ordinal scale, or a 50% reduction in a symptom severity index? Recent RCTs of IBS treatments employ a binary response to a statement about "adequate relief of abdominal pain and discomfort" or "satisfactory relief of IBS symptoms."

A primary outcome measure may be the intensity of a single symptom, a global outcome measure that embraces several salient symptoms, integration of symptoms into a numerical index, or the summary score of a symptom severity/frequency questionnaire. Other measures might comprise a reduction in symptoms below a predefined threshold. A frequently used scale called the *Irritable Bowel Symptom Severity Scale* attempts to assess severity, but for symptoms like pain or bloating such measures do little more than record frequency, duration, and effects on daily living. Ordinal and VAS rating scales are reproducible and sensitive to change but cannot compare an individual's symptom severity to that of another. A meaningful clinical response must be defined beforehand, so that the patients who achieve it can be identified as responders.

FGIDs do not alter life expectancy, but they may affect quality of life (QOL). A measure of the impact of an FGID treatment on health-related quality of life (HRQOL) is often a secondary outcome variable in FGID RCTs. Examples of validated HRQOL instruments include the *Sickness Impact Profile* and *the SF-36 (Short Form of the General Health Questionnaire)*. Disease-specific QOL questions examine the impact of a particular disease on quality of life and include problems specific to that disease (e.g., the fear of fecal incontinence in IBS). An example is the *IBS-QOL*. HRQOL measurements are subject to a subject's mood and personality, which impairs their usefulness as primary outcome measures. An optimistic, outgoing person will respond more positively to a QOL question than someone who is introverted, depressed, or anxious. Such human diversity confounds disease specificity and remind us of the complex biopsychosocial nature of patients—indeed of us all.

Analysis and Reporting

The CONSORT statement, first published in 1996, aims to improve the quality of RCT reporting. CONSORT guidelines emphasize the importance of clearly reporting why the study was undertaken and how it was carried out and analyzed. It includes a twenty-two-item checklist (table 15-3). A flowchart (figure 15-2) describes how patients progress through a study. It consists of four sections: *Enrollment, Allocation, Follow-up, and Analysis*. Adherence to these guidelines improves trial methodology and the quality of data reporting. Many medical journals require that reports of RCTs conform to CONSORT guidelines. (www.consort-statement.org.)

The type of statistical analysis to be used for a trial will be determined by

Table 15-3. CONSORT Checklist of Items to Report in a Randomized Trial

REPORT SECTION AND TOPIC	DESCRIPTOR
Title and Abstract	How participants were allocated to intervention, (e.g, "random allocation")
Introduction, Background	Scientific background and rationale
Methods	
Participants	Eligibility criteria for participants; settings and locations where data were collected
Interventions	Precise details of interventions intended for each treatment group and how they were administered
Objectives	Specific objectives and hypotheses
Outcomes	Defined primary and secondary outcome measures and methods that were used to enhance the quality of measurements (e.g., multiple observations, training of assessors)
Sample size	How sample size was determined
Randomization	
Sequence generation	Method used to generate the random allocation sequence, including details of any restrictions
Allocation concealment	Random allocation sequence (e.g., numbered containers or central telephone); how sequence was concealed until the interventions were assigned
Implementation	Who generated the allocation sequence, who enrolled participants, who assigned participants to their groups
Blinding (masking)	Were participants, those administering the interventions, and those assessing outcomes blinded to group assignment?
Statistical methods	How the success of blinding was evaluated; statistical methods that were used to compare groups for primary outcome(s) and subgroup analyses

REPORT SECTION AND TOPIC	DESCRIPTOR
Results	
Participant flow	Flow of participants through each stage; numbers of participants randomized, receiving intended treatment, completing study protocol, and analyzed for the primary outcome; protocol deviations from the study plan
Recruitment	Dates of recruitment and follow-up
Baseline data	Baseline demographic and clinical characteristics of each group
Numbers analyzed	Number of participants (denominator) included in each analysis. Was analysis "intention-to-treat"? State results in absolute numbers (e.g., 10/20, not 50%).
Outcomes and estimation	For each primary and secondary outcome, a summary of each group's results, with 95% confidence intervals
Ancillary analyses	Other analyses, including subgroup analyses and adjusted analyses; indicate if prespecified or exploratory
Adverse events	All important adverse events or side effects
Comment	
Interpretation	Interpretation of the results, accounting for study hypotheses, potential bias or imprecision, and dangers associated with multiple analyses and outcomes
Generalizability	Generalizability of the trial findings
Overall evidence	Interpretation of the results in the context of current evidence

Adapted from *Rome III: The Functional Gastrointestinal Disorders,* pp. 812-813.

Figure 15-2. CONSORT flow diagram to indicate participant progress through the four phases of a clinical trial. (Adapted from *Rome III: The Functional Gastrointestinal Disorders*, p. 811.)

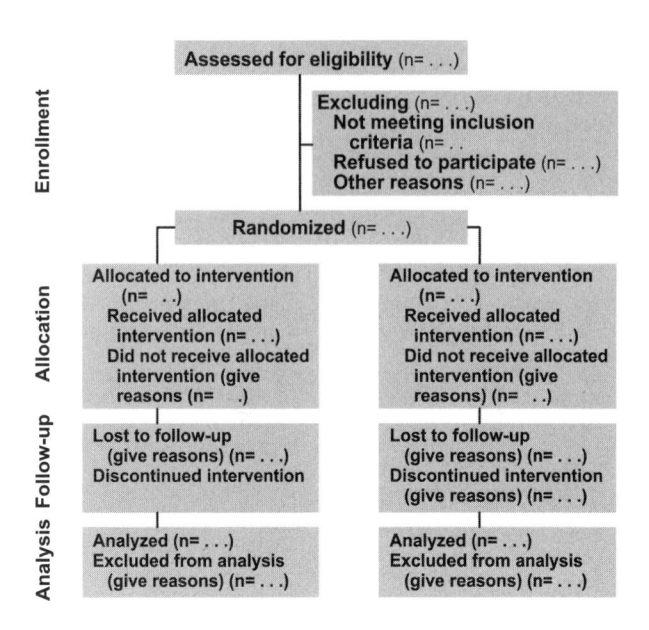

the study design and the primary outcome measure upon which the overall conclusion is based. The difference between active and placebo treatments should be accompanied by 95% two-sided confidence intervals (as opinion polls would state it, "correct nineteen times out of twenty"). Expression of statistically significant differences between study groups should state the actual *P* value (e.g., *P* = .04). The reciprocal of the therapeutic gain in a treatment efficacy trial (1/ therapeutic gain) computes the number of like patients who need to be treated (NNT) in order to encounter one who will experience a clinical benefit. The number needed to harm (NNH) is similarly calculated. A so-called type I statistical error occurs when data analysis indicates a positive result when none exists. The type I error rate may be inflated by multiple comparisons. When you ask enough questions a positive reply is inevitable. The *Bonferroni correction* derives a new *P* value by dividing the original by the number of outcomes.

Statistical analysis should be based on an intention-to-treat (ITT) principle where dropouts are considered to be nonresponders. Per-protocol analysis (all patients receiving treatment after randomization) may be biased unless the reasons for dropping out are known.

Ethical Issues

It is misleading and unethical if the original primary outcome measure is abandoned for another in order to favor a treatment. Subgroup analysis or secondary analysis of data not predicted in the original hypothesis are purely exploratory. Unpublished negative treatment trials are often omitted from reviews of multiple trials—the result is that the remaining favorable trials overestimate treatment efficacy and underestimate adverse events. Therefore, investigators have an obligation to publish their data, regardless of the outcome. Many medical journals require prior entry of RCTs in a publicly accessible trial registry. It is likely that regulatory agencies will adopt a similar position.

Randomized Clinical Trials and Evidence-based Medicine: A Perspective

Like a poem, a clinical trial can never be perfect. Given the ambitions of the investigators, the humanity of the trial subjects, and the beliefs of physicians who must use the data, much can go wrong between the hypothesis and the consulting room. Although the RCT is the best tool we have for evaluating treatments, we should briefly consider its advantages and limitations.

Advantages

Randomized controlled trials prove the efficacy of treatments and tests. In addition, they provide early warning of harmful effects that otherwise may be unnoticed. If a drug is useful, mild adverse effects like nausea may be tolerable, but more severe effects such as liver damage and untoward interactions with other drugs are unacceptable. Clinical trial evidence should lead to the removal of useless or harmful treatments from the formulary. This protects patients and saves money. The process of discarding old tests and treatments is more difficult than it should be; RCTs for older treatments would make the task easier.

Some complain that RCTs delay access to valuable new treatments. This complaint is untenable—science cannot be rushed. Were the treatment known to be useful, there would be no need for a trial. Ineffective treatments waste money and risk harm. In the 1950s, the drug thalidomide was prematurely released for treating nausea during pregnancy and caused tragic birth deformities. Some people worry that control patients in RCTs are denied the benefits of the test treatment. This worry is unjustified, for those on treatment may fare no better, or even worse.

By scientifically scrutinizing disease, patients, and treatments, trial investigators can learn more about them. Sometimes, there is an unexpected result that leads to new knowledge unanticipated by the investigators. Like Alexander Fleming's fortuitous contamination of a bacterial culture with penicillin mold, many important medical discoveries are serendipitous.

Some RCT benefits are less tangible. They improve confidence in medical treatments. Participants learn more about their illnesses and get excellent care. Clinical trials results are the scientific basis of medicine and the core of its reputation.

Limitations

Clinical trials have shortcomings, to be sure. Even when they are carefully conducted, they may produce falsely negative results (type II errors). Flawed entry criteria, frequent dropouts, or an inappropriate outcome measure may weaken a trial result's applicability to patients. More disturbing is the possibility that a false-positive result legitimizes a useless therapy (type I error). Unless we subject falsely categorized treatments to retrial, or to careful postmarketing follow-up, the truth may never be known.

Trial results provide little guidance on the optimal dose of a drug for an individual. Instead, the physician must adjust the dose according to the patient's age, size, and possibly a physiologic measure such as the blood sugar or pulse. Choosing an incorrect dose of the test drug for an RCT may result in failure to show benefit or unacceptable side effects.

The cost of bringing a drug from conception to regulatory approval is $800 million over a decade, and clinical trials are the most costly component. This expense may inhibit the development of new drugs, especially where the potential for sales is small. More worrying is the bias towards new prescription drugs, while other or older treatments often are neglected. Only a pharmaceutical firm can undertake a large RCT, and then only if it foresees a profit.

The flip side of expensive trials for new drugs is that most treatments are untested. Who will sponsor the necessary clinical trials for inadequately tested drugs, diets, procedures, and alternate therapies? Occasionally, a treatment controversy spurs individual investigators to undertake small, inexpensive, but valuable clinical trials, and granting agencies may support them. Nevertheless, many older treatments remain at large without ever having their efficacy and safety established. Is it not an irony that we know so much about the merits and demerits of new drugs through RCTs involving thousands of patients, yet other commonly used medical and alternative treatments are submitted to no such scrutiny?

Meta-analyses and Systematic Reviews

Often several clinical trials of a treatment have conflicting outcomes or insufficient data to yield a conclusion. Where the entry criteria, outcome measures, and trial conduct are similar, it is fashionable to combine the data from such trials in search of a definitive answer. Regrettably, these conditions are seldom true in FGID trials. Several existing meta-analyses and systematic reviews of IBS treatments are unsatisfactory because of the flawed and heterogenic nature of the existing trials. Such armchair exercises add little to our knowledge of FGID therapy. FGIDs need more hands-on, independent, and properly conducted RCTs.

Conclusion

Some discoveries such as renal transplantation and coronary angioplasty dramatically demonstrate medical treatments whose benefits are self-evident. Randomized clinical trials cannot compete with these for public acclaim. Nevertheless, RCTs are one of the most important clinical developments of the twentieth century. They are the only means for new drugs to be approved in Western countries, and they increasingly validate other treatments as well. Even transplantation and angioplasty require validation in subsets of patients to ensure that they are efficaciously and safely deployed. Nevertheless, most treatments—especially those for the FGIDs—are inadequately tested. Ideally, RCTs using the *Rome III* guidelines should be applied to all putative FGID treatments. Then, and only then, could these disorders truly be managed by evidence-based medicine—a worthy but probably impossible ideal. Meanwhile, we must make do with the scant existing evidence, the accumulated wisdom, the general measures (chapter 13), and the known positive effects of the placebo effect and time (chapter 14). These enable an informed choice from among the more specific treatments that are discussed next.

Sources

Begg C, Cho M, Eastwood S, Horton R, Moher D, Olkin I, Pitkin R, et al. Improving the quality of reporting of randomized controlled trials. The CONSORT statement. *JAMA*. 1996;276(8):637-639.

Camilleri M, Chey WY, Mayer EA, Northcutt AR, Heath A, Dukes GE, McSorley D, Mangel AM. A randomized controlled clinical trial of the serotonin type 3 receptor antagonist alosetron in women with diarrhea-predominant irritable bowel syndrome. *Arch Intern Med*. 2001;161:1733-1740.

Irvine EJ, Whitehead WE, Chey WD, Matsueda K, Shaw M, Talley NJ, van Zanten SV. Design of treatment trials for functional gastrointestinal disorders. In: Drossman DA, Corazziari E, Delvaux M, Spiller RC, Talley NJ, Thompson WG, Whitehead WE, eds. *Rome III: The Functional Gastrointestinal Disorders*. McLean, VA: Degnon Associates, Inc.; 2006:779-833.

Mueller-Lissner SA, Fumagalli M, Bardhan KD, Pace F, Pecher E, Nault B, Rüegg P. Tegaserod, a 5-HT4 receptor partial agonist, relieves symptoms in irritable bowel syndrome patients with abdominal pain, bloating and constipation. *Aliment Pharmacol Therap*. 2001;15:1655-1666.

Thompson WG. *The Placebo Effect: Combining Science and Compassionate Care*. Amherst, NY: Prometheus Books; 2005.

16 Management of the Functional Gastrointestinal Disorders

Introduction
So far, we have addressed the general measures that should apply to the treatment of all the functional gastrointestinal disorders (FGIDs), and have illustrated the importance of a good therapeutic relationship to successful outcomes. This chapter discusses the treatments that are promoted for each disorder; some of them are described with more detail in chapter 17. These treatments are not meant to be everyone's prescription, but rather a menu from which doctors and patients may choose. To that end, we briefly discuss the medical evidence supporting them. First however, we should consider how doctors and patients—and third-party payers—should make their choices.

Which is the Best Treatment?
Every patient with an FGID should benefit from the general measures outlined in chapter 13. For many patients—probably most of those in primary care—diagnosis, empathy, education, prognosis, and reassurance are sufficient. Others, especially those referred to specialists, require more. Because there is no reliable FGID cure, any treatment must be considered to be palliative. How then should one choose from the treatments outlined in this chapter? One size does not fit all! The choices should take into account the diagnosis, prognosis, need for treatment, evidence that the treatment works, adverse effects, and availability.

A diagnosis of globus or proctalgia fugax seldom justifies specific treatment because the symptoms are short-lived and usually produce no disability. However, if the diagnosis were functional dyspepsia or irritable bowel syndrome, where symptoms impair work or quality of life, palliation is desirable. These chronic disorders may begin in youth and last a lifetime, so the emphasis should be on lifestyle and coping mechanisms rather than indefinite drug therapy. If drugs are used, they should be prescribed for a few weeks and, if successful, repeated only as needed. In contrast, a socially devastatingly disorder like fecal incontinence warrants more aggressive therapy.

Given the great variety of feelings and behaviors among humans, only patient and doctor can decide whether a treatment is needed, and determine how much and for how long. Some action is necessary when one's ability to do one's job or socialize are impaired and general treatment measures fail. As a general rule, palliation should be on an as-needed basis. Drugs should target the most prominent symptom in doses and treatment periods that minimize adverse events. The symptoms of any FGID may be intolerable by themselves, but we should be mindful of the somatic and psychological comorbidity that frequently accompany them. Some FGID symptoms will not likely improve with treatments that are directed solely at the gut. In some anorectal disorders and severe IBS, psychological treatments such as biofeedback or cognitive behavioral therapy may produce lasting improvement in a person's ability to cope with the symptoms.

One should choose the treatment best supported by evidence. Ideally, the characteristics of the patient and his disorder should resemble those subjects from whom the evidence was gathered. If evidence is lacking, the treatment should be at least plausible—there should be a scientific hypothesis to explain its possible utility. Complementary and alternative therapies and even much time-worn medical advice may be implausible as well as unproven.

The FGIDs have good prognoses in the sense that, although they are often incurable, they do not predispose to death or physical disability. Therefore, treatments with significant adverse effects are usually unacceptable. For severely affected people, some risk may be acceptable, but only after its full disclosure. This philosophy explains the temporary withdrawal of the drugs alosetron and tegaserod by the U. S. Food and Drug Administration and their subsequent approval for restricted use.

Finally the treatment should be locally available. Few circumstances justify seeking care far from a local physician who should know the patient best. Some treatments are unevenly available. For example, hypnotherapy for IBS is common in Europe, while cognitive behavioral therapy is practiced mainly in North America. Other centers concentrate on psychotherapy or biofeedback. The drug alosetron is available only in the United States. Tegaserod is available in several countries including parts of Latin America. It was widely used in the United States, but now is available only with special arrangements. It remains unapproved in Europe. Table 16-1 illustrates the diverse approvals of drugs for IBS. These differences are largely due to the drugs' history, the local marketing efforts of manufacturers, and each nation's concern over cost and safety. We should ponder whether a drug's lack of regulatory unanimity is a sign of uncertainty about its efficacy.

Table 16-1. Drugs Officially Approved for IBS in Five Western Countries

Generic Name	Trade Name	Action
Australia		
Dicyclomine	Merbentyl	Anticholinergic
Alverine	Alvercol	Papaverine-like
Mebeverine	Colese, Colofac	Antispasmodic
Peppermint oil	Mintec	Carminative
Propantheline	Pro-Banthine	Anticholinergic
Canada		
Dicyclomine	Bentylol	Anticholinergic
Propantheline	Pro-Banthine	Anticholinergic
Hyoscyamine	Levsin	Anticholinergic
Scopolamine N-butylbromide	Buscopan	Anticholinergic
Pinaverium	Dicetel	Calcium channel blocker
Trimebutine	Modulon	Kappa opiate antagonist
France		
Prifinium	Riabal	Anticholinergic
Alverine	Spasmaverine	Papaverine-like antispasmodic
Mebeverine	Colopriv, Duspatalin	Antispasmodic
Pinaverium	Dicetel	Calcium channel blocker
Trimebutine	Modulon, Transacalm	Kappa opiate antagonist
Hyoscyamine sulfate	Sulfate de Duboisine	Anticholinergic
UK		
Hyoscine butylbromide	Buscopan	Anticholinergic
Dicyclomine	Merbentyl	Anticholinergic
Alverine	Spasmonal	Papaverine-like antispasmodic
Mebeverine	Colofac	Antispasmodic
Peppermint oil	Colpermin, Mintec	Carminative
Propantheline	Pro-Banthine	Anticholinergic
USA		
Hyoscine methobromide/ methscopolamine bromide	Pamine	Anticholinergic
Dicyclomine	Bentyl	Anticholinergic
Hyoscyamine sulfate	Levsin	Anticholinergic
Hyoscyamine, atropine	Donnatal, Barbidonna	Anticholinergic
Scopolamine hydrobromide	Scopace	Antispasmodic
Propantheline	Pro-Banthine	Anticholinergic
Alosetron	Lotronex*	5-HT$_3$ antagonist
Tegaserod	Zelnorm*	5-HT$_4$ partial agonist

*Restricted use
From Thompson WG and Heaton KW, 2003. Updated with the assistance of Blair Jarvis, Clinical Editor, Canadian Pharmacists Association, and Kristin McCulloch, Pharmacy Student, University of Toronto.

continues

Sources For Table 16-1.
Index Nominum. International Drug Directory, 18th ed. Swiss Pharmaceutical Society, eds. Stuttgart: medpharm GmbH Scientific Publishers, 2004.
Martindale: The Complete Drug Reference, 35th ed. Sweetman SC, ed. London: Pharmaceutical Press, 2007.
American Hospital Formulary Service Drug Information 2007. McEvoy GK, ed. Bethesda, MD: American Society of Health System Pharmacists, 2007.
Government of Canada. "Health Canada," Drug Product Database, http://www.hc-sc.gc.ca/dhp-mps/prodpharma/databasdon/index_e.html (accessed July 2007).
Government of Australia, Department of Health and Ageing. "PBS (Pharmaceutical Benefits Schedule) for Health Professionals," http://www.pbs.gov.au/html/healthpro/home (accessed July 2007).
BMJ Publishing Group Ltd and RPS Publishing, "British National Formulary 53," http://www.medicinescomplete.com/mc/ (accessed July 2007).

TREATMENTS FOR THE FGIDS

In this section we review the treatments that have been proposed for the individual disorders and the evidence supporting them. The choice of treatments should be made with a physician's advice. Dosages and manner of administration can be found in the *Rome III* book or standard texts. Citations are available in the *Rome III* book and supplemented in the sources listed at the end of this chapter. In the following sections, trade names for patented drugs are included once only. More details about some of the treatments are found in the next chapter.

A. FUNCTIONAL ESOPHAGEAL DISORDERS

The most common esophageal symptom is heartburn due to gastroesophageal reflux disease (GERD), which is usually promptly relieved by a proton pump inhibitor (PPI). Sometimes, esophageal chest pain and dysphagia are also due to GERD. Thus, the first order of therapy of presumed functional esophageal disorders is to try maximum doses of a PPI.

A1. Functional heartburn

Patients with heartburn and no alarm symptoms should undergo at least a trial of acid suppression with a PPI or histamine$_2$ (H$_2$) receptor antagonist. These drugs relieve heartburn due to acid reflux whether or not there is esophagitis. Patients with functional heartburn will not respond because acid reflux appears not to be the cause of their symptoms. Indeed, a diagnosis of functional heartburn in practice depends upon the heartburn's failure to improve on PPI therapy (chapter 10).

Functional heartburn patients who are unresponsive to PPIs have few treatment options, none of which have been evaluated by satisfactory randomized controlled trials (RCTs). Some patients may be offered a trial of antidepressants such as low-dose tricyclic antidipressants or selective serotonin reuptake inhibitors (SSRIs). Others may undergo behavioral modification or relaxation therapy. If reflux of nonacid gastric contents is convincingly demonstrated to cause functional heartburn, antireflux measures such as upright posture and prokinetic drugs may help.

A2. Functional chest pain of presumed esophageal origin

Management begins with exclusion of cardiac, extraesophageal, and esophageal disease. Patients who have the noncardiac nature of their pain explained to them use fewer health resources and improve their work. However, such reassurance rarely abolishes a patient's concern, and spontaneous recovery is rare.

There are few drug options. Functional chest pain excludes GERD. Nevertheless, all patients should try a PPI at maximum dose. So-called "smooth-muscle relaxants" such as calcium channel blockers (e.g., *nifedipine*) and anticholinergics (e.g., *dicyclomine*) seem ineffective, which is not surprising since esophageal smooth-muscle contractions apparently do not cause the pain. *Botulinum toxin* injected into the lower esophageal sphincter reduces chest pain in some subjects, most of whom have a (probably irrelevant) esophageal motor disorder. In these reports a placebo effect is possible, indeed likely, since the data are uncontrolled.

Transcutaneous electrical nerve stimulation (TENS) may relieve functional chest pain of presumed esophageal origin. One placebo-controlled study showed TENS reduced sensitivity to intraesophageal balloon distention in patients with unexplained chest pain.

The most encouraging treatments are psychopharmacologic drugs and behavioral interventions. Antidepressants appear to relieve pain independent of any effect on depression, anxiety, or esophageal function. They may also improve sleep, reverse autonomic dysregulation or somatization, and block stress effects in the cerebral cortex. Low doses of the antidepressant *trazodone* bring global improvement and reduce distress in patients with chest pain and spastic esophageal motility disorders. Relief is unrelated to any motility change. In addition, the tricyclic antidepressant *imipramine* is superior to placebo. The recommended doses are less than those used for psychiatric disorders. An eight-week RCT of *sertraline*, a selective serotonin reuptake inhibitor (SSRI), also improved chest pain. Antidepressants relieve uncomfortable emotional symptoms that compromise a person's ability to cope.

Behavioral therapy may help patients with functional chest pain. One technique includes relaxation training with controlled diaphragmatic breathing exercises. In a trial of education, controlled breathing, relaxation training, and diversion of attention from pain, patients with chest pain experienced fewer chest pain episodes, greater functional capacity, and lessened psychological distress. An eight-week trial of cognitive behavioral therapy (CBT) in patients with chest pain reduced chest pain episodes and improved anxiety and depression scores, disability ratings, and exercise tolerance. CBT alone was superior to usual care in another study of unexplained chest pain. Small numbers of patients and poorly disguised controls such as "waiting list" or "usual care" weaken these studies. The improvements may be placebo.

A3. Functional dysphagia

The management of functional dysphagia requires reassurance that there is no obstruction, the avoidance of precipitating factors, careful chewing of food, and psychological care. As for functional chest pain, PPI therapy should be tried in all patients, but terminated if ineffective and if there is neither reflux nor esophagitis. Functional dysphagia may improve over time, and overzealous treatment is unwarranted. Nevertheless, patients with more severe symptoms should have therapeutic trials of smooth-muscle relaxants, anxiolytics, or antidepressants.

Passing a mechanical dilator to stretch the esophagus may temporarily improve intermittent dysphagia, especially if an esophageal stricture or ring has been overlooked, or if the dysphagia is associated with a spastic motor disorder. *Botulinum toxin* injections are sometimes tried, but have a transient benefit at best.

A4. Globus

After the symptom is determined *not* to be dysphagia, patients with globus need reassurance that no serious disease is present and there are no dire consequences. If there is associated heartburn, or other evidence of GERD, a short-term PPI trial might be tried, but antacids are unlikely to relieve globus itself. The results of small, poorly controlled trials of other antacid drugs and prokinetics do not support their use for this long-term, minor complaint.

B. FUNCTIONAL GASTRODUODENAL DISORDERS
B1. Functional dyspepsia

The available data are based on studies of functional dyspepsia prior to *Rome III*. None exists regarding the treatment of the newly described epigastric pain syndrome (EPS) or postprandial distress syndrome (PDS). Despite careful history-taking, some dyspepsia patients may actually have GERD. As a result, randomized trials of antacid and antisecretory drugs in dyspepsia may inadvertently yield misleading data.

DIET
Coffee and other caffeine drinks may aggravate symptoms and consumption should be moderated. Stopping smoking and reducing alcohol consumption are good ideas even if abstinence fails to relieve dyspepsia. Aspirin and nonsteroidal antiinflammatory drugs (NSAIDs) cause dyspepsia and should be stopped when practical, or covered by antacid or antisecretory drugs. Anecdotal reports suggest that avoiding spicy and fatty foods may lessen postprandial dyspepsia. Because fat slows stomach emptying, six small, low-fat meals per day may decrease early satiety, postprandial fullness, bloating, and nausea. These plausible suggestions are untested by RCTs.

MEDICATION
Antacid and antisecretory medications. Although many patients with functional dyspepsia take antacids such as calcium carbonate (TUMS), the practice is not supported by RCTs. However, subjects who respond to these over-the-counter medications are unlikely to participate in clinical trials, so their effectiveness cannot be dismissed. A Cochrane meta-analysis of eleven of H_2-receptor antagonists in functional dyspepsia reports them superior to placebo. The estimated number needed to treat (NNT) is 8—a modest indication of efficacy. However, some of the included small trials misclassify GERD as functional dyspepsia. Another Cochrane meta-analysis of seven placebo-controlled, randomized trials of PPIs in functional dyspepsia also reports efficacy with an NNT of 7. Effectiveness appears to be independent of dose, but again some GERD patients may be included in the reviewed trials.

Eradication of H. pylori infection. Yet another Cochrane meta-analysis reports a 9% improvement of dyspepsia one year after *H. pylori* eradication compared to placebo (NNT = 15). A further meta-analysis reported no significant benefit, but omitted some trials. A patient might prefer not to risk the adverse effects of antibiotics for such an uncertain benefit.

Prokinetics. Metoclopramide is prokinetic drug that stimulates gastric emptying and gut peristalsis. In poor-quality studies, it appears to be efficacious in functional dyspepsia. Most studies are equivalence trials and not placebo-controlled. Metoclopramide has rare, but serious cardiac and neurological adverse effects that should limit its use for benign dyspeptic symptoms. The actions of *domperidone* (Motilium) resemble those of metoclopromide. It improves symptoms in patients with functional dyspepsia without speeding up gastric emptying. A meta-analysis indicates that domperidone is superior to placebo against dyspepsia. However, it may cause breast symptoms and is unavailable in the United States. *Cisapride* is a serotonin 5-HT_4 agonist and 5-HT_3 antagonist that activates cholinergic motor neurons to stimulate upper gut peristalsis. In dyspepsia, two meta-analyses of cisapride compared with placebo demonstrated that it relieves epigastric pain, early satiety, abdominal distention, and nausea. Publication bias may partly account for the positive results. Because of rare fatal cardiac arrhythmias, cisapride is now unavailable in most countries. *Tegaserod* (Zelnorm) is a partial 5-HT$_4$ agonist that increases preprandial and postprandial gastric volumes, which suggests that it may reduce fullness in functional dyspepsia. Early trials show no significant benefit over placebo. *Erythromycin* is a macrolide antibiotic that increases the gastric emptying rate in patients with diabetic and idiopathic gastroparesis (stomach paralysis), but there are disadvantages of using an antibiotic for a chronic functional disorder. Erythromycin and similar macrolide compounds may produce intolerable abdominal cramps and diarrhea.

Other drugs. There are one positive and one negative trial of *sucralfate* (Sulcrate) in functional dyspepsia. *Bismuth* (DeNol), previously used in Europe to treat peptic ulcers, is inadequately tested in functional dyspepsia. The anticholinergic drug *dicyclomine* (Bentyl, Bentylol) was no better than placebo in relieving symptoms of dyspeptic patients in two small crossover studies. Likewise, a double-blind crossover trial showed *trimebutine* (Modulon) to be no better than placebo in dyspepsia. Therefore, use of these drugs to treat functional dyspepsia has no rationale. Antidepressants may be useful in difficult cases, especially if the patient is depressed.

Dyspepsia subtypes

Dyspepsia subtypes derive from the notion that certain patients with dyspepsia have unique mechanisms that may be amenable to drug therapy. Their existence as distinct entities is yet to be verified. The epigastric pain syndrome (EPS) should respond to pain medication. Since antidepressants are useful in chronic pain, they may prove useful here. PPIs have also been used with mixed success. The postprandial distress syndrome (PDS) may be due to either delayed gastric emptying or incomplete receptive relaxation of the upper part of the stomach. It may therefore respond to prokinetic drugs for the former, or medications that relax gastric tone for the latter, such as tegaserod or buspirone. Criteria proposed to identify these possibly drug-responsive subtypes are found in appendix A.

PSYCHOTHERAPY AND HYPNOTHERAPY

In one trial, psychotherapy was superior to supportive therapy in improving dyspepsia after twelve weeks, but there was no difference at one year. An uncontrolled study found that hypnotherapy improved symptoms and quality of life in patients with functional dyspepsia, and reduced their subsequent use of medications.

COMPLEMENTARY AND ALTERNATIVE MEDICINE

One controlled trial reports improved dyspepsia during treatment with herbal preparations that contained extracts from bitter candy tuft, matricaria flower, peppermint leaves, caraway, licorice root, and lemon balm. However, how herbal medicines act and which components are active remain mysteries. Furthermore, their stability and concentration differ from product to product. Ginger root appears effective for nausea and vomiting, and has some properties including prokinetic activity that may make it useful in dyspepsia. Preliminary acupuncture and acupressure data are not encouraging.

B2. Belching disorders
(B2A. AEROPHAGIA AND B2B. UNSPECIFIED EXCESSIVE BELCHING)

Explanation of the symptoms and reassurance that belching does not mean disease are important. It is useful to demonstrate a patient's forceful chest expansion that sucks in air before each belch. If the habit is not too established, aerophagia can be unlearned through behavioral techniques or antianxiety medications. Stress reduction or treatment of associated psychiatric disease may help as well. Some doctors advise against sucking hard candies or chewing gum, and encourage eating slowly with small swallows. Avoiding carbonated beverages seems obvious, but carbon dioxide, unlike other swallowed gases, is quickly absorbed into the blood and expired rather than belched. Simethicone and activated charcoal preparations are usually ineffective. Sedatives or relaxants may lessen severe aerophagia, but chlordiazepoxide drugs such as *diazepam* (Valium) can habituate, and should be used only for short periods.

B3. Nausea and vomiting disorders
B3A. CHRONIC IDIOPATHIC NAUSEA (CIN)

The 5-HT$_3$ antagonist drug *ondansetron* controls nausea and vomiting during cancer chemotherapy and postoperative care. The mechanism is unknown. *Diphenhydramine* and other histamine$_1$ antagonist, anti–motion-sickness drugs affect the middle ear rather than the gut. Their sedative effects may help, or they may induce unacceptable drowsiness. It is uncertain if either drug improves CIN.

B3B. FUNCTIONAL VOMITING

Vomiting patients may develop nutritional deficiencies or dehydration that must be corrected. Tricyclic antidepressants are sometimes used in low or full doses. Mirtazepine may have selective effects on some patients with nausea. Antiemetic drugs induce drowsiness and seldom help.

B3C. CYCLIC VOMITING SYNDROME (CVS)
Severe attacks of cyclical vomiting may require hospital admission to maintain hydration and nutrition. Antimigraine medications are used, especially if family members have migraine headaches. Serotonin (5-HT$_1$) agonists such as *sumatriptan* (Imitrex) can be given by mouth, subcutaneous injection, or nasal spray, but are contraindicated in ischemic heart disease, stroke, and uncontrolled hypertension. Beta blockers help some people. A tricyclic antidepressant (*amitriptyline, doxepin, nortriptyline*) or an SSRI (*fluoxetine*) may at least improve the cyclic vomiting patient's mood. A new implanted "gastric stimulator" activates the vagal nerve to reduce nausea and vomiting.

B4. Rumination syndrome in adults
PPIs suppress any coexisting heartburn and protect the esophageal mucosa, but do little for rumination itself. Behavioral modification called "habit reversal" uses breathing techniques to suppress the urge to regurgitate. Rumination and breathing exercises cannot be performed simultaneously.

C. FUNCTIONAL BOWEL DISORDERS
C1. Irritable bowel syndrome (IBS)
The type and severity of symptoms and associated psychosocial issues determine the treatment. Most patients respond to general measures, a strong physician-patient relationship, and a multicomponent treatment approach. The physician should maintain contact with the patient and avoid overtesting or harmful treatments. Patients should beware of nutrition-depleting diets and have regular, unhurried meals. Dietary fiber for IBS with constipation is time-honored, inexpensive, and safe, but poorly substantiated by clinical trials. Indeed, some patients claim bran exacerbates their symptoms. The only substantial randomized controlled trial of bran in IBS suggested it exacerbated flatulence and did not relieve pain.

MEDICATION
Early therapeutic trials had substantial methodological inadequacies, and a publication bias undermines most systematic reviews. No treatment addresses the complete IBS syndrome. Therefore, drug therapy should be directed toward the dominant symptom(s). *Loperamide* (Imodium) may prevent diarrhea when taken before a meal or before an important social or business occasion. Constipation, not IBS itself, often responds to dietary fiber supplements such as whole wheat bran, up to three tablespoons per day. If not, commercial fiber products containing psyllium (ispaghula) may help. However, neither fiber nor loperamide has been found helpful for IBS pain.

A group of pharmacologically unrelated drugs dubbed "smooth-muscle relaxants" address the notion of colon spasm. They are the most commonly used

IBS drugs, but their usefulness is unsubstantiated by most clinical trials. In some cases, therapeutic doses produce significant side effects. Several systematic reviews seem to support the use of this group of drugs, but the reviews' reliability is compromised by the drugs' dissimilarity, the faulty trials chosen for review, and the aforementioned publication bias. Based on the available data none would achieve regulatory approval today.

Antidepressants help more severely affected patients even in the absence of psychiatric comorbidity. The recommended lower-than-antidepressant dose minimizes side effects. Analysis of data from controlled trials is hampered by a high dropout rate, but a per-protocol analysis of one otherwise well-designed study achieved an NNT of 4 with *desipramine*. Desipramine showed no significant benefit over placebo in an intention-to-treat analysis, but did show statistically significant benefit in the per-protocol analysis, especially when participants with nondetectable blood levels of desipramine (indicating lack of treatment compliance) were excluded. This tricyclic antidepressant seems to improve symptoms in women with moderate-to-severe IBS irrespective of dose, providing they adhere to the drug program. The SSRI *paroxitine* is less effective for pain, but improves the quality of life in patients with severe IBS. It achieves better global improvement than a high-fiber diet.

Alosetron (Lotronex), a selective serotonin $5\text{-}HT_3$ receptor antagonist, slows gut transit and provides adequate relief in women with diarrhea and IBS according to large, well-conducted clinical trials (NNT = 7). *Tegaserod* (Zelnorm), a partial $5\text{-}HT_4$ receptor agonist, improved a different global outcome measure in women with IBS and constipation. (NNTs for 12 mg and 4 mg daily were 14 and 20). However, the principle benefit appears to derive from its laxative effect. Recent data support its use in men as well as women. Both drugs have had regulatory difficulties due to possible adverse events: ischemic colitis and severe constipation with alosetron, and coincidence with cardiovascular complications with tegaserod. In the United States, these rare events led first to withdrawal, then reintroduction with restricted access. Neither drug is approved by the European Union, but tegaserod is available in many countries in Asia and Latin America. Lubiprostone is one of a new class of agents called chloride channel activators. It has been approved for use in chronic constipation, and preliminary studies indicate that it also has benefit in relieving the pain and constipation of IBS. This drug has been submitted for approval by the U.S. Federal Drug Administration for IBS with constipation.

CHANGING THE BACTERIAL FLORA

In preliminary trials, probiotics improve IBS symptoms, possibly by altering the composition of the bacterial flora from "bad" to "good" bacteria. In the only well-controlled study, patients taking *Bifidobacterium infantis* fared better than those on placebo and had reduced inflammatory substances in the bowel. Larger randomized trials of this and other probiotics are needed. Some authors blame small-bowel bacterial overgrowth, diagnosed by a lactulose-hydrogen breath test. Antibiotics may be helpful in a very small proportion of patients with IBS if there is associated bacterial overgrowth. However, they may provide only transient benefit. Their use risks *Clostridium difficile* superinfection, allergic reactions, and antibiotic resistance. One agent (Rifaximin) is locally active in the GI tract. More proof of efficacy is needed before exposing IBS patients to the risk of antibiotic treatment.

PSYCHOLOGICAL AND BEHAVIORAL TREATMENT

Cognitive-behavioral therapy, standard psychotherapy, or hypnotherapy may help selected, severely-affected IBS patients. Drossman and colleagues (2003) conducted a single-blind twelve-week trial of CBT that yielded a 70% improvement in global satisfaction and quality of life (not pain) compared with 37% with weekly educational sessions. Multicomponent treatment, including behavioral therapy, may be more effective than medical therapy alone. Hypnotherapy, which normalizes rectal sensation, is the most thoroughly evaluated psychological treatment for IBS. Twelve sessions benefitted quality of life, anxiety, and depression in previously refractory patients, and the benefits appeared to last at least five years. Compared with usual care, eight sessions of individual psychotherapy can improve quality of life and reduce health care costs. However, controlled trials of the psychological therapies cannot be fully double-blind, and the treatments are time-consuming, costly, and available only in certain locales. If the treatment is successful, the benefit is prolonged.

C2. Functional bloating

Most bloating research is done on patients who have the symptom as part of IBS or other FGID. Treatment is similar whether bloating occurs alone or as part of another disorder. Bloating is not necessarily accompanied by excess intestinal gas, so proposed gas-reducing treatments may miss the mark. Rather, it may be due to increased sensitivity of the nerves in the intestinal tract or abnormal relaxation of the abdominal wall muscles, producing distension.

DIET

When a patient bloats after eating dairy products (not yogurt), fresh fruits, or juices, a suspicion of lactose or fructose intolerance might warrant further investigation or dietary exclusion. However, even lactase-deficient patients can tolerate small amounts of milk, and restriction should not compromise calcium or vitamin intake. Avoiding flatulogenic foods such as beans or bran, exercising regularly, losing excess weight, and taking activated charcoal are recommended by some doctors, but with neither rationale nor supporting evidence.

MEDICATION

The surfactant *simethicone* reduces bloating in some studies but not others. Antibiotics are risky and unlikely to help, but trials of probiotics are encouraging. *Beano*, an over-the-counter oral enzyme solution that digests glucose linkages in complex carbohydrates, reduces flatus but not bloating. *Pancreatic enzymes* reduce the bloating, gas, and fullness due to a high-calorie, high-fat meal. *Tegaserod* improves bloating in some female IBS patients with constipation, according to randomized trials where bloating is a secondary outcome measure.

C3. Functional constipation

Patients who fear that failure to evacuate for two or three days is harmful should be reassured that daily defecation is not essential. Regular visits to the toilet, increased fluid intake, and physical exercise are recommended. Some physicians suggest that patients assume the "squat position" on the toilet by raising the feet with a footstool. Occasionally, constipation is cured by discontinuing a constipating medication or treating depression. Treatment should be guided by the severity of the symptoms and, if necessary, the results of physiological tests that are discussed under defecation disorders (below and table 7-2).

FIBER SUPPLEMENTATION AND BULK LAXATIVES

Most patients with mild-to-moderate constipation respond to increased dietary fiber ingestion, which should be aggressively tried and proven ineffective before proceeding to other treatments. Fiber increases fecal weight, intestinal transit, and stool frequency. Experiments with plastic "stools" indicate that less effort is required to expel large stools than small ones. Increased fecal weight due to wheat fiber and psyllium (ispaghula) is dose-dependent and requires a week to reach a steady state. The laxative effect probably depends upon intestinal distension by the increased volume of water and bacteria, and the production of laxative, short-chain fatty acids. Coarse bran is more effective than fine bran, perhaps due to tactile stimulation of the intestinal mucosa. Insoluble products like wheat bran or whole-grain foods, or soluble-fiber bulk laxatives (e.g., psyllium products, methycellulose), or any combination are safe and usually effective if taken adequately and regularly. However, insoluble fiber products may produce more bacterial fermentation and a feeling of gaseousness.

Increasing one's dietary fiber intake is difficult, so daily fiber supplements of up to three tablespoonsful of bran may be required. However, patients may complain of flatulence, distension, bloating, and a disagreeable taste. Those with defecation disorders or slow transit respond poorly. A number of commercial bulking agents are available over the counter. Psyllium is available as a powder or in capsules. A common trade name is Metamucil, but there are many cheaper generic preparations. Methylcellulose (Citrucel) is also available in powder or capsule form. A third alternative to bran is *polycarbophil* (Konsyl, Equalactin). All of these products are unabsorbed from the intestine; they bulk the stool by attracting water. Because they swell when wet, they should be taken with at least eight ounces of water to avoid choking.

LAXATIVES

When the above measures have been adhered to and fail, patients turn to laxatives. Most commercial laxatives have adverse effects if abused, and should be chosen with care, especially by the elderly or patients with renal impairment. Excessive use may deplete electrolytes such as sodium and potassium. Surprisingly few randomized trials have evaluated laxatives. Several classes are described in chapter 17. Most laxatives are available over the counter and are safe if used according to directions on the package. Milk of magnesia, an osmotic laxative, and bisacodyl, a stimulant, represent safe options for mild constipation.

Serotonin (5-HT) influences gastrointestinal motility, secretion, and sensation. 5-HT_4 receptor agonists are prokinetic serotonin analogues that stimulate the peristaltic reflex and accelerate gastrointestinal transit. Tegaserod, a selective, partial 5-HT_4 receptor agonist, is superior to placebo for patients with chronic constipation (NNT = 8 with 6 mg bid). Di Palma and colleagues report the first comparison trial of tegaserod with a laxative, *polyethylene glycol* (PEG). The PEG appears to be superior and cheaper. This result needs confirmation but it highlights an important principle. Other than the Di Palma data, no randomized trials permit us to judge tegaserod's efficacy and safety compared to less costly laxatives.

A new agent, *lubiprostone* (Amitiza), a prostaglandin analogue, is approved in the United States and Japan for chronic constipation, but not in Europe, Australia, or Canada. No comparative trials with tegaserod or other laxatives have yet been performed. Lubiprostone replaces an earlier prostaglandin E_1 analogue, *misoprostol* (Cytotec). It does not appear to risk abortion, as does misoprostil, but because it has not been properly tested in pregnancy, it probably should be avoided by women who are pregnant or may become pregnant.

An enema's volume stimulates defecation and may be necessary for severe constipation due to disordered defecation. Phosphate enemas (Fleet) distend the colon and have osmotic effects as well.

C4. Functional diarrhea

If a careful history and examination suggest functional diarrhea, the diagnosis should be explained to the patient at the first consultation. Understanding normal gut physiology and how diet, stress, and/or low-grade inflammation might accelerate colonic transit is helpful, as is the reassurance that the symptoms are unlikely to develop into serious disease. The prognosis of functional diarrhea is uncertain, especially if the stool weight exceeds 500 grams. Many patients with chronic idiopathic diarrhea appear to either recover or acquire a treatable organic diagnosis after about three years.

Wheat bran, vegetables, and fruit fibers should be decreased, and some physicians advocate a low-residue diet. Drinks containing caffeine, sorbitol, or mannitol should be kept to a minimum. Some patients with functional diarrhea benefit from fructose exclusion. With a dietician supervising to prevent nutritional deficiencies, attention to diet helps patients contribute to their own management.

Opioids are the principle drug treatments for diarrhea, and *loperamide* is the best tolerated. This drug increases anal tone, slows gut transit, and is not considered a narcotic. It controls diarrhea and reduces urgency and stool frequency in IBS with diarrhea (NNT = 1.2). The dose is adjusted as necessary. Alternatively, loperamide may be taken in anticipation of a stressful social or work engagement. An alternative, *diphenoxylate* (Lomotil), contains atropine. Codeine, tincture of opium, and other narcotics are effective, but not ideal for chronic diarrhea.

The 5-HT$_3$ antagonist alosetron is effective in some women with IBS and diarrhea (NNT = 7), and was recently shown to benefit men. It slows transit and reduces the gastrocolonic response in normal people, but there are no published RCTs in patients with functional diarrhea. *Cholestyramine*, a powdered resin, binds bile salts and prevents their laxative effect. It is sometimes effective in functional diarrhea. Bile salt absorption is measured by ingestion of the isotope Se^{75}HCAT that is later measured in the breath. Some physicians simply try cholestyramine and skip the test.

D. FUNCTIONAL ABDOMINAL PAIN SYNDROME (FAPS)

General measures for treating FAPS include those discussed in earlier chapters, with some special considerations. Because some patients hold unrealistic expectations for rapid improvement or cure, the physician must place the prognosis in perspective. Realistic treatment goals are symptom relief, improved daily function, and rehabilitation—but not cure. Regular visits reinforce these goals.

MEDICATION

Tricyclic antidepressants relieve chronic pain and depression. Rare randomized trials in FAPS and extrapolation from RCTs in other painful FGIDs suggest that low doses can improve both visceral and somatic pain. If necessary, the dose may be increased and augmented with psychological treatments. Unfortunately, some patients poorly adhere to therapy because of side effects and fear of stigmatization. Adherence is better if the patient understands that antidepressants have analgesic properties in other painful diseases like migraine, postherpetic neuralgia, and diabetic neuropathy. If side effects are intolerable, a serotonin-norepinephrine reuptake inhibitor also helps pain. Benefit may take several weeks, but side effects fortunately also diminish with time.

When symptoms are more severe, two treatments can be combined to maximize benefit and minimize side effects. Treatment combinations include combining a low-dose tricyclic with an SSRI, an antidepressant with the anxiolytic *buspirone*, or an antidepressant with a psychological treatment. Benzodiazepines such as *diazepam* (Valium) should be avoided because of their potential for dependency and abuse. Moreover, they may lower pain thresholds and exacerbate symptoms.

Most analgesics (e.g., aspirin and NSAIDs) are unhelpful, probably because their actions are peripheral and the pain is central in origin. The chronic use of narcotics risks addiction and a narcotic bowel syndrome that is characterized by impaired gut motility and increased pain sensitivity.

PSYCHOLOGICAL THERAPY

A diary describing the circumstances of the pain and their emotional and cognitive responses helps patients to share responsibility for their care, and helps their physicians to gain insight into aggravating factors and how patients cope. If patients connect intermittent pain episodes to psychological distress, they may respond to psychological treatments. Some may be reluctant to see a mental health specialist because they fail to understand the benefit. Others feel stigmatized or see referral as a rejection. The analgesic effects of tricyclic antidepressants may help such patients accept psychotherapy later. A mental health professional can help patients manage the pain and reduce psychological distress while medical care continues.

There are no randomized trials of psychological treatments for FAPS, but studies in other painful conditions suggest such treatments might be beneficial. CBT identifies maladaptive thoughts, perceptions, and behaviors, and develops ways to increase symptom control. Dynamic or interpersonal psychotherapy seeks to reduce psychological distress and physical symptoms that are exacerbated by difficult interpersonal relationships. Stress management aims to counteract the physiological effects of stress or anxiety. Multidisciplinary pain clinics manage chronic pain patients with comprehensive care, rehabilitation, and narcotic withdrawal.

OTHER INTERVENTIONS

Spinal manipulation and massage for FAPS lack supportive RCTs. Data for acupuncture are scarce in chronic pain management and nonexistent for FAPS. TENS is likewise of uncertain value. Nerve blockade designed for peripheral pain is inappropriate because the locus of the pain is central. Adhesions are scars binding intestinal segments together that result from previous abdominal surgery or infection that are thought (usually erroneously) to cause abdominal pain. A randomized trial of one hundred patients with chronic abdominal pain compared laparoscopic cutting of adhesions to laparoscopy alone, and unsurprisingly the results were the same.

E. FUNCTIONAL GALLBLADDER AND SPHINCTER OF ODDI (SO) DISORDERS

Examination and some treatments of the functional biliary disorders require invasive endoscopic procedures that explore the biliary tree. Complications such as pancreatitis or a tear in the bile duct are so severe that endoscopic retrograde cholangiopancreatography (ERCP) is recommended only in patients with severe and disabling biliary pain who fulfill the *Rome III* criteria. If there are no gallstones or other pathology, endoscopic surgery of the biliary tree should be considered *only* in those who fulfill criteria for the functional SO disorders and are unresponsive to nifedipine or tricyclic antidepressants. Investigation and treatment should be undertaken in properly equipped centers with experienced and expert personnel. A second opinion before proceeding is wise.

E1. Functional gallbladder disorder

The treatment of this disorder is cholecystectomy if there are recurrent episodes of moderate-to-severe biliary pain and gallbladder emptying is impaired. Neither the natural history of this functional disorder, nor whether it causes an inflamed gallbladder, is known. Treatment with gallstone-dissolving ursodeoxycholic acid is not indicated because there are no gallstones.

E2. Functional biliary SO disorder

Nitroglycerine and the calcium channel blocker *nifedipine* decrease SO pressure, but side effects occur in up to one-third of patients. *Botulinum toxin* injected into the sphincter reduces sphincter pressure and improves bile flow for a few months. There are no controlled or long-term studies of these therapies. Balloon dilation of the SO has unacceptable complications, primarily pancreatitis, so endoscopic sphincterotomy is the most widely used therapeutic procedure. Cutting the sphincter through the endoscope during ERCP is cheaper, cosmetically preferable, and safer than open surgery. In two randomized trials, patients with removed gallbladders and functional biliary SO disorder were improved after sphincterotomy at two and four years compared to those having sham sphincterotomy. A third RCT favorably compares endoscopic sphincterotomy with open surgery.

E3. Functional pancreatic SO disorder

Drugs fail to ameliorate this rarely documented disorder. Recurrent pancreatitis due to SO dysfunction is treated by cutting the biliary and pancreatic SO to permit free bile and pancreatic juice flow into the duodenum. This should be done only in patients when endoscopic manometry demonstrates an elevated SO basal pressure. To facilitate drainage of bile and pancreatic juice, a stent (small tube) may be left in the duct temporarily.

F. FUNCTIONAL ANORECTAL DISORDERS
F1. Functional fecal incontinence

Diarrhea is a strong risk factor for fecal incontinence. Constipation (if it involves fecal impaction in the rectum) may also cause fecal incontinence. The rational use of drugs to improve an incontinent patient's bowel habit requires an accurate stool description. The Bristol Stool Form Scale may help (figure 6-1). In those with diarrhea (Bristol types 6 and 7) and incontinence, fiber supplementation may normalize stool consistency enough to prevent incontinence. If fiber fails, taking *loperamide* thirty minutes before meals improves diarrhea and slightly increases internal sphincter tone. In patients with both constipation and diarrhea, the drug must be given in such a way as to reduce diarrhea, yet avoid constipation. Loperamide before social occasions helps incontinent patients prevent embarrassing accidents and gain confidence. *Diphenoxylate*, combined with *atropine* (Lomotil) is less effective than loperamide and has more side effects. The serotonin 5-HT$_3$ antagonist *alosetron* also may be used to treat diarrhea-related fecal incontinence. Patients with constipation (Bristol types 1 and 2), fecal impaction, and overflow incontinence may benefit from an evacuation program that incorporates combinations of regular manual evacuation, bisacodyl or glycerine suppositories, fiber supplementation, and/or oral laxatives. An alternative is an osmotic laxative such as lactulose, 10 ml twice daily, with an enema weekly.

Biofeedback addresses two contributing causes of fecal incontinence: weakness of pelvic floor muscles and/or decreased rectal sensation (i.e., decreased ability to sense the presence of stool in the rectum, which is a cue that tells the patient when to contract pelvic floor muscles to prevent incontinence). Training employs a balloon in the rectum to simulate rectal filling and sensors in the anal canal to detect contraction of the pelvic floor muscles. Assisted by tracings of balloon distention and anal pressure that are transmitted to a monitor, incontinent patients learn to contract the external anal sphincter when they feel the balloon distending. The procedure is repeated with progressively smaller volumes until the patient can manage alone. Although an RCT in 2003 failed to show that computer-assisted biofeedback was better than advice and verbally taught pelvic-floor exercises, a subsequent study demonstrated that biofeedback was significantly more effective than education and medical management, and more effective than pelvic-floor exercises. Patients with severe sensory impairment and those with major structural defects or complete denervation of the pelvic floor are less likely to benefit from biofeedback training, but those with milder defects do well with this treatment.

Anal sphincter repair for functional fecal incontinence is disappointing. *Sacral nerve stimulation* through a device implanted at the base of the spine

160 Understanding the Irritable Gut

augments anal pressures and improves continence. This technique is the subject of a current multicenter study. The last resort is colostomy, where feces are diverted through an opening of the bowel and abdominal wall into a bag that is emptied at the patient's convenience.

F2. Functional anorectal pain
F2A. CHRONIC PROCTALGIA
(F2A1. LEVATOR ANI SYNDROME AND F2A2. UNSPECIFIED FUNCTIONAL ANORECTAL PAIN)

Treatments of these disorders aim to reduce tension in the striated (voluntary) pelvic floor muscles. They include electrogalvanic stimulation, biofeedback, digital massage of the levator ani muscles, and sitz baths. Muscle relaxants such as *methocarbamol, diazepam,* and *cyclobenzaprine* also have been tried. None of these treatments has been shown to be effective in controlled trials. One randomized trial indicates that intrasphincteric injection of *botulinum toxin* is no better than placebo in levator ani syndrome. If treatment is deemed necessary, it is safe to select one of the above because they are without significant adverse consequences. In contrast, surgical procedures cannot correct this functional disorder and may cause incontinence. Chronic proctalgia is a chronic pain syndrome and some of the measures described under FAPS may be appropriate.

F2B. PROCTALGIA FUGAX

Proctalgia fugax is harmless, unpleasant, and incurable. For most patients, pain episodes are so brief that treatment is impossible, and so infrequent that prevention is impractical. The treatment is reassuring explanation. For the few severely affected patients who have attacks that last at least twenty minutes, one randomized trial showed that inhalation of *salbutamol* (a beta adrenergic agonist) shortened the attacks more than placebo.

F3. Functional defecation disorders

Dyssynergic defecation (F3a) refers to inability to relax pelvic floor muscles during attempted defecation. Inadequate defecatory propulsion (F3b) refers to failure to contract abdominal wall muscles sufficiently when straining to defecate. Three randomized controlled trials show biofeedback to be more effective for these disorders than laxatives, placebo, sham biofeedback, or standard care. Training involves three steps:

1. Teaching the patient to strain by providing feedback on rectal pressure or abdominal wall contraction.
2. Teaching pelvic floor relaxation by applying sensors to the anus to provide feedback on voluntary anal muscle contraction and relaxation.

3. Simulated defecation, where the patient practices evacuating an artificial stool.

Approximately 70% of patients with functional defecation disorders are successfully treated with biofeedback. However, success depends upon the skills of the biofeedback therapist; experienced practitioners are limited to a few academic medical centers. Laxatives are less effective than biofeedback but may be the only treatment available to some patients.

Conclusion

This chapter presents the treatments recommended for the FGIDs. Further information and citations can be obtained in *Rome III: The Functional Gastrointestinal Disorders,* chapters 7 through 12. Some treatments are discussed in more detail in the next chapter. No therapy suits every FGID patient. Rather, physicians and patients should select from those available, taking into account the medical evidence and the patient's needs and preferences.

Sources

Behar J, Corazziari E, Guelrud M, Hogan WJ, Sherman S, Toouli J. Functional gallbladder and sphincter of Oddi disorders. In: Drossman DA, Corazziari E, Delvaux M, Spiller RC, Talley NJ, Thompson WG, Whitehead WE, eds. *Rome III: The Functional Gastrointestinal Disorders.* McLean, VA: Degnon Associates, Inc.; 2006:595-635.

Camilleri M, Bueno L, De Ponti F, Fioramonti J, Lydiard RB, Tack J. Pharmacological and pharmacokinetic aspects of functional gastrointestinal disorders. In: Drossman DA, Corazziari E, Delvaux M, Spiller RC, Talley NJ, Thompson WG, Whitehead WE, eds. *Rome III: The Functional Gastrointestinal Disorders.* McLean, VA: Degnon Associates, Inc.; 2006:161-229.

Chiarioni G, Bassotti G, Stegagnini S, Vantini I, Whitehead WE. Sensory retraining is key to biofeedback therapy for formed stool fecal incontinence. *Am J Gastroenterol.* 2002;97:109-117.

Chiarioni G, Whitehead WE, Pezza V, Morelli A, Bassotti G. Biofeedback is superior to laxatives for normal transit constipation due to pelvic floor dyssynergia. *Gastroenterology.* 2006;130:657-664.

Creed F, Levy RL, Bradley LA, Drossman DA, Francisconi C, Naliboff BD, Olden KW. Psychosocial aspects of the functional gastrointestinal disorders. In: Drossman DA, Corazziari E, Delvaux M, Spiller RC, Talley NJ, Thompson WG, Whitehead WE, eds. *Rome III: The Functional Gastrointestinal Disorders.* McLean, VA: Degnon Associates, Inc.; 2006:295-267.

Di Palma JA, Cleveland MV, McGowan J, Herrera JL. A randomized, multicenter comparison of polyethylene glycol laxative and tegaserod in treatment of patients with chronic constipation. *Am J Gastroenterol.* 2007;102(9):1964-1971.

Drossman DA. Treatment for bacterial overgrowth in the irritable bowel syndrome. *Ann Intern Med.* 2006;145(8):626-628.

Drossman DA, Toner BB, Whitehead WE, Diamant NE, Dalton CB, Duncan S, Emmott S, et al. Cognitive-behavioral therapy versus education and desipramine versus placebo for moderate to severe functional bowel disorders. *Gastroenterology.* 2003;125:19-31.

Galmiche JP, Clouse RE, Bálint JA, Cook IJ, Kahrilas PJ, Paterson WG, Smout AJPM. Functional esophageal disorders. In: Drossman DA, Corazziari E, Delvaux M, Spiller RC, Talley NJ, Thompson WG, Whitehead WE, eds. *Rome III: The Functional Gastrointestinal Disorders.* McLean, VA: Degnon Associates, Inc.; 2006: 369-417.

Heymen S, Scarlett Y, Jones K, Ringel Y, Drossman D, Whitehead WE. Randomized, controlled trial shows biofeedback to be superior to alternative treatments for patients with pelvic floor dyssynergia-type constipation. *Dis Colon Rectum.* 2007;50:428-441.

Johanson JF, Morton D, Geenen J, Ueno R. Multicenter, 4-week, double-blind, randomized, placebo-controlled trial of lubiprostone, a locally-acting type-2 chloride channel activator, in patients with chronic constipation. *Am J Gastroenterol.* 2008;103(1):170-177.

Longstreth GF, Thompson WG, Chey WD, Houghton LA, Mearin F, Spiller RC. Functional bowel disorders. In: Drossman DA, Corazziari E, Delvaux M, Spiller RC, Talley NJ, Thompson WG, Whitehead WE, eds. *Rome III: The Functional Gastrointestinal Disorders.* McLean, VA: Degnon Associates, Inc.; 2006: 487-555.

Norton C, Chelvanayagam S, Wilson-Barnett J, Redfern S, Kamm MA. Randomized controlled trial of biofeedback for fecal incontinence. *Gastroenterology.* 2003;125:1320-1329.

Rao SS, Seaton K, Miller M, Brown K, Nygaard I, Stumbo P, Zimmerman B, Schulze K. Randomized controlled trial of biofeedback, sham feedback, and standard therapy for dyssynergic defecation. *Clin Gastroenterol Hepatol.* 2007;5:331-338.

Spiller R. Clinical update: irritable bowel syndrome. *Lancet.* 2007;369(9573): 1586-1588.

Tack J, Talley NJ, Camilleri M, Holtmann G, Hu P, Malagalada J-R, Stanghellini V. Functional gastroduodenal disorders. In: Drossman DA, Corazziari E, Delvaux M, Spiller RC, Talley NJ, Thompson WG, Whitehead WE, eds. *Rome III: The Functional Gastrointestinal Disorders.* McLean, VA: Degnon Associates, Inc.; 2006:419-485.

Thompson WG, Heaton KW. *Fast Facts: Irritable Bowel Syndrome*, 2nd ed. Oxford: Health Press; 2003.

Wald A, Bharucha AE, Enck P, Rao SS. Functional anorectal disorders. In: Drossman DA, Corazziari E, Delvaux M, Spiller RC, Talley NJ, Thompson WG, Whitehead WE, eds. *Rome III: The Functional Gastrointestinal Disorders.* McLean, VA: Degnon Associates, Inc.; 2006:639-685.

17 Treatments

Introduction

In the last chapter we discussed the more specific treatments for the functional GI disorders (FGIDs) that have been published in *Rome III: The Functional Gastrointestinal Disorders*. This chapter contains further information about the most important of these, including their modes of action and their adverse effects.

Drugs

Antacid and Antisecretory Drugs

Some antacid drugs have been in use for a century, but potent ones are of more recent vintage. They relieve heartburn due to gastroesophageal reflux disease (GERD). Proton pump inhibitors (PPIs) are the most effective and are of interest here because in practice their failure to relieve symptoms is a prerequisite for diagnosis of the functional esophageal disorders. Because antacid drugs were also the principal treatments for peptic ulcer disease, it was natural that they also be tried for functional dyspepsia where the symptoms are similar. However, unlike heartburn, the medical evidence for their efficacy in dyspepsia is modest, and may depend upon the presence of GERD among dyspepsia trial participants.

Antacids. When stimulated, the stomach's parietal cells produce a gastric fluid pH of less than 2. A pH of 7 is neutral, and that of cell fluids is about 7.3. Antacids relieve the symptoms of peptic ulcer and heartburn by neutralizing gastric acid and raising the pH towards 7. Antacids may be no better than placebo in treating functional dyspepsia. However, they are safe, inexpensive, and available over the counter, so patients often try them before consulting a physician. Most commercially available antacids are combinations of aluminum and magnesium hydroxide. Calcium carbonate (TUMS) is also popular. Some weak effervescent antacids contain sodium bicarbonate, known as baking soda. Antacids are usually flavored and some contain the "antiflatulent" *simethicone*. This surfactant breaks up bubbles within the gut, presumably rendering gas available for absorption, but its clinical effectiveness is unproven.

For heartburn, an antacid combined with *alginate* (Gaviscon) is designed to float on stomach fluids and protect the esophagus from acid exposure.

H_2 antagonists. Before the PPIs appeared in the late 1980s, the histamine (H_2) antagonists were the preferred peptic ulcer and heartburn treatments; they remain among the world's largest selling drugs. Analagous to the action in the nose of the H_1 antihistamines in hay fever, H_2 antagonists compete with histamine for receptors on the gastric parietal cells to inhibit acid secretion. They are very safe and effective for heartburn and are available over the counter at half the prescription dose. H_2 antagonists are commonly used for functional dyspepsia too, with less impressive results.

Four commercially available H_2 antagonists are *cimetidine, ranitidine, nizatidine,* and *famotidine*. Their patents are mostly expired, and generic trade names vary. These H_2 blockers differ in potency, but there is little to choose among them for efficacy and safety. They may interfere with the metabolism of some drugs, notably warfarin and theophyllin. Cimetidine sometimes causes confusion in the elderly.

Proton pump inhibitors (PPIs). In gastric parietal cells, the proton pump comprises the enzyme *hydrogen, potassium adenosine triphosphatase* (H+, K+ - ATPase) that "pumps" hydrogen ions into the stomach, acidifying its contents. A family of drugs known as the *benzimidazoles* irreversibly incapacitates this enzyme. Even in modest doses, these drugs (actually prodrugs) are the most powerful known inhibitors of gastric acid secretion. The concentration of the benzamidazoles in the parietal cells is so great that their half-life in the blood is about an hour. At an acid pH, PPIs bind with sulphydryl groups on the H+, K+ - ATPase to permanently inactivate the enzyme. However, new acid pumps are continuously synthesized and about a third of the stomach's acid secretory capacity is restored 36 hours after a single dose. Nevertheless, if taken regularly, even modest doses almost completely block acid production.

Omeprazole (Losec, Prilosec), *lansoprazole* (Prevacid), *pantoprazole* (Pantozol), *rabeprazole* (Pariet) and *esomeprazole* (Nexium) are available in most countries, and there are few important differences among them. Their principal uses are the management of GERD, the protection of the upper gut during the administration of NSAIDS, and (combined with antibiotics) the eradication of *H. pylori*. Adverse effects of PPIs are unusual, but profound acid suppression risks enteric infections, especially travellers' diarrhea, *Clostridium difficile,* and bacterial overgrowth in the small intestine.

Other antiulcer drugs. Sucralfate (Sulcrate) forms a protective barrier over a peptic ulcer. One would not expect it to work in functional dyspepsia because there is no ulcer to protect. *Misoprostol* (Cytotec) is a prostaglandin with laxative properties, also of uncertain efficacy. *Bismuth citrate* (DeNol), a European antiulcer drug with some anti-*H. pylori* activity, shows merely a trend towards improved dyspepsia. None of these is now commonly used.

Eradication of H. pylori

The reclusive organism *Helicobacter pylori* lurked unnoticed in the stomach lining until Warren and Marshall discovered in the mid 1980s that it caused chronic gastritis and gastric and duodenal ulcers—an observation that earned them the Nobel Prize. We have since learned that if these organisms can be eradicated from the stomach of someone with gastritis, the gastritis will heal and that person will no longer be liable to a peptic ulcer (unless caused by an NSAID). After many trials, physicians have learned that full doses of a PPI twice daily for a week combined with two antibiotics will achieve eradication in most patients. This is an astonishing achievement when we recall that duodenal ulcer was the most common reason for army discharge in World War II. The antibiotics most frequently chosen are *clarithromycin* with either *amoxicillin* or *metronidazole*, along with a PPI. However, these combinations are changing as greater antibiotic resistance is occurring. The good news is that the frequency of *H. pylori* infection causing ulcer disease is decreasing. The interest here is that some patients with functional dyspepsia also have *H. pylori*, and the pressure (not the evidence) to kill it is very strong.

Prokinetics

Prokinetics are a diverse group of drugs that enhance stomach emptying of solids and fluids and the propulsive activity of the intestines. Because slow gastric emptying causes bloating and postprandial fullness in patients with neuromuscular diseases of the stomach such as gastroparesis, prokinetics are prescribed to FGID patients who have similar symptoms. However, their effectiveness is difficult to validate. In gastroesophageal reflux disease (GERD), they are recruited when PPIs fail, or if the refluxing gastric contents are not acid.

The original prokinetic, *metoclopramide* (Reglan, Maxeran), releases acetylcholine from cholinergic motor neurons in the gut wall, thereby stimulating propulsion. Unlike others, metoclopromide crosses the blood-brain barrier where its dopamine-stimulating activity causes neurologic side effects that include anxiety, drowsiness, hallucinations, confusion, odd posturing (dystonia), a tremor resembling Parkinson's disease, and an irreversible disturbance called tardive dyskinesia. Metaclopromide may prolong the QT interval in the electrocardiogram, which indicates a risk of cardiac arrythmias. Diarrhea and breast enlargement in males are other disadvantages. Nevertheless, sedating, antinausea, and antivomiting effects make the drug useful for cancer patients who are made ill by chemotherapy. Because of its potentially adverse events, it should be used cautiously, if at all, for functional gut disorders.

Domperidone (Motillium) is a peripheral dopamine antagonist that promotes gastroduodenal coordination. This drug differs from metoclopramide and cisapride in that it is not cholinergic and does not enter the central nervous system, so that neurological adverse effects are fewer. Its antinausea and antivomiting effects are mediated through the so-called chemoreceptor trigger zone at the base of the brain, but outside the blood-brain barrier. Dopamine is a neurotransmitter that through the enteric nervous system delays gastric emptying. Domperidone, by antagonizing dopamine, speeds up gastric emptying. Because it increases lower esophageal sphincter (LES) tone, some physicians recommend it for GERD. It may help prevent reflux in patients at risk of aspiration. Like other prokinetics, some trials indicate benefit in functional dyspepsia. However, these are flawed and affected by publication bias. Domperidone occasionally causes painful breasts in men and lactation in women due to increased secretion of the pituitary hormone prolactin. It is unavailable in the United States.

Cisapride (Propulsid) is a substituted benzamide that, unlike domperidone and metoclopramide, does not affect the dopamine system. In the gut myenteric plexus, it releases acetylcholine—a neurotransmitter that increases motor activity throughout the gut. Cisapride increases gastric antral contractions and favors gastroduodenal coordination. It also increases LES pressure and promotes small bowel and colon motility, so its therapeutic profile is similar to that of domperidone. It has been a second-line drug for GERD treatment, but its efficacy in dyspepsia and other functional disorders is likely nil. Cardiac arrythmias forced this drug off the market in many countries; efforts continue to find a safer drug with cisapride's favorable characteristics.

The macrolide antibiotic *erythromycin* causes annoying cramps and diarrhea due to faster gastric emptying and shorter gastrointestinal transit. These side effects are potential assets if a prokinetic effect is required. The macrolide effect is mediated through smooth-muscle receptor sites for the gut hormone motillin, which activates intestinal migrating motor complexes and peristalsis. Erythromycin may be tried in dyspepsia for now, but the pharmaceutical industry is examining new macrolides that stimulate gut motility without antibiotic affects.

Another prokinetic, tegaserod, stimulates intrinsic serotonin receptors. See "Serotonin Analogues" below.

"Smooth-Muscle Relaxants"

The hypothesis that colon spasm causes irritable bowel (IBS) symptoms is nearly two centuries old; the disorder is still sometimes called the "spastic" colon. This belief is unsupported by data, but underlies the notion that so-called smooth-muscle-relaxing drugs, sometimes called antispasmodics, should relieve IBS and other FGID symptoms. Drugs with anticholinergic properties such as *atropine* and the quaternary ammonium compounds have been tested in the treatment of IBS since the 1940s, with no convincing evidence that they are effective. (Some studies in the 1970s suggested that anticholinergics reduce pressure in the intestines after eating, but this observation did not correlate with symptom improvement.) Nevertheless, more recent systematic reviews and meta-analyses combine the published trials of several drugs that relax gut smooth muscle in order to validate their use in IBS. The reviewers include such diverse drugs as anticholinergics (*dicyclomine, cimetropium, octilium, hyocyamine*), a smooth-muscle relaxant (*mebeverine*), a calcium channel blocker (*pinavarium*), an opiate antagonist (*trimebutine*), and peppermint oil, which makes their conclusions problematic since these drugs have disparate modes of action. Publication bias is likely since the unpublished and presumably negative trials of pharmaceutical companies are omitted. Unsuccessful trials of older antispasmodics such as propantheline are also missing. M_3 muscarinic antagonists, an α_2 adrenergic agonist, and an opiate antagonist each failed to demonstrate gut-relaxing efficacy sufficient for regulatory approval, yet they too are omitted from the reviews.

Based on commonly recognized guidelines for IBS trials (Klein 1988), and on the statements of the authors of the reviews themselves, almost all the reviewed studies are flawed. Trial entry criteria are seldom stated, and only very recent studies employ symptom criteria. Many trials include subjects without pain, and one review permits a trial's inclusion if "at least 51% of subjects had IBS." Outcome measures and endpoints (three days to twenty-four weeks) differ from trial to trial. Often, neither was a primary outcome stated beforehand, nor was an adjustment made for multiple outcomes. Crossover trials are included, despite their inappropriateness for fluctuating conditions like IBS.

In recent years, none of these so-called smooth-muscle relaxants have been submitted for approval to North American or European regulatory authorities for the treatment of IBS, since supporting data are not forthcoming. Over thirty years ago, based upon physiological, rather than clinical evidence, the U. S. Food and Drug Administration deemed anticholinergics like dicyclomine as "possibly effective" for the treatment of IBS. Some smooth-muscle relaxants are approved by some national regulatory authorities and not by others (table 16-1), perhaps inspiring further skepticism. Nevertheless, regulatory-grandfathered anticholinergics are the most commonly prescribed drugs for IBS in the United States.

The smooth-muscle relaxants, particularly the anticholinergics, have side effects ranging from dry mouth to urinary retention. Physicians and patients must decide if the evidence and risks justify a course of such a drug. If so, the medication should be taken for symptom episodes rather than on a chronic basis. The symptoms should be carefully monitored and the drug withdrawn if there is no improvement.

Serotonin Analogues

Serotonin (5-HT) is an important neurotransmitter in the brain and the gut. Many psychoactive drugs, such as the selective serotonin reuptake inhibitors (SSRIs), act to alter serotonin activity in the brain. There are at least twelve serotonin receptors distributed throughout the body; many are found in the intestines. Hence, research focused on gut serotonin activity led to several drugs that inhibit or augment certain receptors, notably the 5-HT$_3$ and 5-HT$_4$ receptors. As noted in chapter 16, *alosetron*, a selective serotonin 5-HT$_3$ receptor antagonist, slows gut transit and provides "adequate relief" in women with diarrhea and IBS according to large, well-conducted clinical trials. Its benefit in men with IBS has only recently been shown. In the United States, ischemic colitis and severe obstipation led to alosetron's withdrawal, however, more recent studies indicate that when properly used for patients with more severe diarrhea, the risk is reduced. It was later reintroduced specifically for IBS patients with severe symptoms of diarrhea, with restricted access and a risk management program. The drug is unavailable elsewhere.

Tegaserod, a partial 5-HT$_4$ receptor agonist, improved a global outcome measure embracing "satisfactory relief" of gut symptoms in women with IBS and constipation. However, the principal and most consistent benefit appears to derive from its prokinetic and laxative effects that speed up small-intestinal transit. In the United States in August 2007, because of possible adverse effects, tegaserod became available only to those without cardiac disease, with restrictions that required a physician to complete a special form and the patient to give informed consent. In April 2008, the drug was further restricted to hospitalized and severely ill patients. Tegaserod is not approved by the European Union, but it remains available in many parts of Asia and South America.

Development of alosetron and tegaserod advanced the science of randomized controlled trials for IBS and set new standards for their application to all the FGIDs. The drugs relieve some IBS patients with predominant diarrhea or constipation, respectively. Useful trials would compare these drugs with conventional antidiarrheals and laxatives to disclose whether they offer advantages that justify their cost. From a scientific perspective these drugs represent important developments in FGID treatments, and their regulatory difficulties should not be permitted to stifle further progress by industry.

Botox

Botulinum toxin is the ultimate muscle relaxant. It inhibits acetylcholine, hence blocking neuromuscular transmission. A product of *Clostridium botulinin*, it is one of the most powerful neurotoxins known; ingestion of toxin-containing preservatives, contaminated through improper canning, causes a usually fatal paralysis. Known to the public as botox, it can be injected into an aging face to remove wrinkles. It appears to take some wrinkles from the gut as well! In achalasia it relaxes the lower esophageal sphincter, which allows food to pass. When injected into the anus of a patient with an anal fissure, it relieves the associated painful muscle spasm. Like a wrinkled face, a spastic gut requires treatment every three to six months. Botox is of interest here for its largely experimental use in functional esophageal chest pain and dysphagia, and in certain functional anorectal disorders. If the dose is carefully calibrated, the only side effect is unwanted paralysis of muscles adjacent to the injection target.

Antidepressants

Two major classes of antidepressants are used to treat the FGIDs. The tricyclics are older and represented by *amitriptyline* (Elavil), *desipramine* (Norpramin), and *nortriptyline* (Pamelor). They have both serotonin and norepinephrine action and improve chronic pain. Their principle disadvantages are anticholinergic and histaminic side effects such as dry mouth, blurred vision, constipation, and urinary hesitancy. This makes the low doses promoted for the FGIDs especially attractive. A newer class of antidepressant comprises the selective serotonin reuptake inhibitors (SSRIs) represented by *paroxatine* (Paxil). They are better tolerated and easier to administer, but more expensive. For treatment of depression they have largely displaced the tricyclics, and they also benefit anxiety and phobias. However they do not relieve pain. The side effects are usually mild nausea, drowsiness, and fatigue. The recent introduction of serotonin norepinephrine reuptake inhibitors SNRIs (e.g., *duloxetine, venlafaxime*) promises some relief of painful FGIDs. This newest class of antidepressants has both serotonin and norepinephrine activity without the tricyclics' side effects. Their main adverse effect is nausea.

Antidepressants, particularly the SSRIs, are most useful in patients with anxiety as well as depression. They relieve emotional symptoms that interfere with global improvement or coping ability. Nevertheless, it is the pain modulation of the low-dose tricyclic antidepressants that makes them useful for the FGIDs. Extrapolating from the pain literature, many physicians recommend them for the functional abdominal pain syndrome (FAPS). A meta-analysis of antidepressant drug trials in the treatment of IBS concludes that they are effective. However, this review suffers flaws similar to those of the "smooth-muscle relaxant" reviews cited above, and the authors admit that the quality of the reviewed studies is poor. For example, on average the reviewed trials entered only forty-three patients and data from studies of five tricyclics and an antiserotonin agent are lumped together. Only eight of the eleven studies deal exclusively with IBS and the selection criteria were inhomogeneous. The anticholinergic side effects of antidepressants risk a loss of blinding that is not acknowledged. Even the authors recognize that it was impossible to know whether the observed benefits (sic) in functional gastrointestinal disorders are independent of their effects on depression. The best evidence of benefit in the FGIDs derives from the trazadone study for chest pain of presumed esophageal origin, and the desipramine data for IBS that were described in chapter 16.

Probiotics

The inhabitants of the human colon are enduring mysteries. Even today we know little of their identity or function, yet colon microorganisms have potential for good or harm. They are our biological partners—without them our colons would be malnourished, sickly, and more susceptible to infections. Bacteria require the colon to immunologically tolerate them, yet the variety of gut organisms is bewildering. Some doctors advocate altering the colon flora to promote health and treat disease.

Probiotics are living microorganisms, which upon ingestion in certain numbers exert health benefits beyond inherent general nutrition. To achieve this benefit, the organisms must be able to attach to human intestinal cells, colonize the human gut, and resist its natural defenses. Earlier research focused on species of *Lactobacilli*, which were used to treat intestinal infections and inflammations such as childhood rotovirus, *Clostridia difficile*, traveler's diarrhea, and inflammatory bowel disease. With such activity, it is inevitable that gastroenterologists should turn to them for the IBS. Early trials were small, poorly or not-at-all controlled, and failed to declare a primary outcome measure. Nevertheless, they suggest that *Lactobacillus* species benefit some IBS patients. One study of primary care IBS patients shows that *Bifidobacter infantis* improves symptoms compared to a strain of *Lactobacillus* or placebo, with no laxative or antidiarrheal effects. This improvement is associated with improved resistance to gut infection. Indeed, recent research shows that there are "good" and "bad" bacteria, the former strengthening the immunity of the bowel wall to infection. Many patients with IBS not only have fewer "good" bacteria, but also have impaired immunity and inflammation in their gut lining. Probiotics augment the good bacteria.

It is intuitive that interactions between the enteric flora and the host may profoundly affect gut function, but we have little idea what these interactions might be. Some experts suggest that probiotics compete with the indigenous flora to produce antimicrobial metabolites or modulate the local immune response to enteric bacteria. Since IBS patients often recall that their chronic symptoms began with acute enteritis, activated inflammatory mediators may cause their gut dysfunction. Might probiotic alteration of the colon flora displace the organisms responsible for inflammation?

In that "dark continent" that is the human colon there seem to be unlimited bacteria species to test. It even may be possible to manipulate the colon flora through certain foods, such as fermented dairy products (yogurt) or grains (prebiotics). Although the studies to date are encouraging and probiotics seem safe, much more information is required to confirm these data, determine which organisms are efficacious, and elucidate their mechanism of action. Not any probiotic will do, it seems. The shelf life of some of the available products is short, so that few viable organisms reach their target colons.

Laxatives

Ingested osmotic laxatives attract water into the intestines. Thus, unabsorbed sugars such as lactulose, mannitol, and sorbitol increase intraluminal volume and stimulate peristalsis. They are then rapidly metabolized by colon bacteria to short-chain fatty acids with further laxative effect. Up to an ounce (30 ml) of lactulose twice a day is effective in mild constipation, but side effects include abdominal cramps and bloating. Sorbitol is cheaper than lactulose and possibly as effective. Glycerin suppositories act osmotically within the anorectum. Saline laxatives such as magnesium citrate, sodium phosphate and disodium phosphate, and magnesium sulphate are incompletely absorbed. Through osmosis, they cause a net flow of water into the small intestine and colon. Polyethylene glycol (PEG) is an oral, isotonic solution that is used to purge the colon for colonoscopy. For constipation, doses smaller than those required for bowel-cleansing are superior to placebo and lactulose for regular use. Since PEG is not absorbed, has low sodium content, and causes no net potassium or sodium absorption or loss, few adverse effects are expected. *Calcium polycarbophil* acts similarly.

Stimulant laxatives include diphenylmethane derivatives, such as *phenolphthalein* (no longer available in many countries), *bisacodyl, sodium picosulfate* (bisacodyl conjugated with sulphate), and conjugated anthraquinone derivatives, such as *cascara sagrada, aloin,* and *senna*. These drugs decrease net water absorption, stimulate motility, and release prostaglandin. In the colon, sodium picosulphate and the anthraquinone derivatives are cleaved by bacteria to active (unconjugated) agents that stimulate enteric nerves. These over-the-counter agents may be abused, risking metabolic consequences. Melanosis coli, a brown discoloration of the colon lining, is a harmless, reversible consequence of prolonged anthraquinone intake that typically disappears within six months of stopping the drug.

Lubiprostone (Amitiza) was approved by the U. S. Food and Drug Administration in 2006 for chronic constipation. Studies have also shown benefit for the pain and constipation of IBS with constipation, but the drug has not yet been approved for this disorder. Lubiprostone is a locally acting chloride channel activator that enhances chloride-rich intestinal fluid secretion without altering sodium and potassium concentrations in the blood. It has not been properly tested in pregnancy, but it is a prostaglandin analogue that does not appear to risk abortion, as does misoprostil.

Psychological Treatments

A variety of psychological therapies are used to treat FGIDs. Research in their efficacy has advanced recently through standardization of the techniques, but it is difficult to identify control groups with an expectation of improvement equivalent to that of the technique being tested. Because trial subjects are usually recruited from academic centers, it is uncertain that the results of an RCT would generalize to a broader patient population. Nevertheless, psychological treatments are helpful to patients who are severely affected by FGIDs, because many of them suffer from anxiety and depression, experience traumatic life events, and have beliefs or learned behaviors that adversely affect outcome.

Cognitive Behavioral Therapy (CBT)

The basis of CBT is social learning theory, which recognizes that behavior is shaped as a result of its social consequences such as increased attention from others or escape from unpleasant tasks. CBT focuses on ways to increase or decrease a particular behavior. Therapists deploy many techniques to address the thoughts, behaviors, and responses that result from their patients' daily interactions. CBT helps IBS patients recognize the role of illness beliefs and behavior in chronic illness, and addresses anxiety and depression. Relaxation and stress management may further reduce anxiety and autonomic arousal.

Drossman and colleagues' large study found CBT to be more effective than an educational intervention in terms of satisfaction, overall symptom relief, and global well-being after three months, but there is little or no difference in pain scores or in health-related quality of life. This CBT study is of patients who were referred to academic centers, but within this group the benefits are independent of the severity of the IBS. The same therapist administered the CBT and the educational package, so it is uncertain if they were delivered with equal enthusiasm. Nevertheless, these findings illustrate that psychological characteristics are important to the global well-being of patients with FGIDs.

Relaxation Training and Biofeedback

Various relaxation or arousal-reduction techniques teach patients to counteract the physiological effects of stress or anxiety. Methods include progressive muscle relaxation training, biofeedback for striated muscle tension, skin temperature, or electrodermal activity, and transcendental meditation or yoga. Progressive muscle relaxation training and electromyogram (muscle electrical activity) biofeedback reduce skeletal muscle tension, decreasing autonomic arousal and feelings of tension or anxiety.

Biofeedback attempts to reduce smooth-muscle activity through images of body function such as skin temperature or rectal pressure. Transcendental meditation and yoga aim to modify both skeletal muscle tension and autonomic arousal indirectly through cognitive focusing techniques. Studies that examine relaxation training show that it reduces gastrointestinal symptoms.

Nine studies indicate that progressive muscle relaxation training combined with CBT is superior to a waiting-list control group or "conventional medical therapy." Only two studies used an active placebo control, and one found the combination to be superior to an educational treatment. Multicomponent behavioral therapy includes IBS education, progressive muscle relaxation, training in illness-related cognitive coping strategies, problem-solving, and assertiveness training. This combination shows greater IBS symptom reduction than symptom-oriented medical treatment.

Dynamic Psychotherapy

Dynamic psychotherapy, or interpersonal psychotherapy, requires a close relationship between patient and therapist, and may require a long first interview that begins with a detailed discussion of bowel symptoms. In this context, phrases such as "I feel all churned up inside" and "I fear losing control" are made in relation to bowel symptoms. Later these phrases can be brought back to the patient who might link them to troublesome aspects of his life. Some FGID patients experience interpersonal problems that may be associated with childhood adversity and difficulty in trusting others. In therapy, these difficulties recur, leading to increased anxiety or distress, often linked to abdominal discomfort. As patients understand their relationship problems they may act upon these insights and thus reduce psychological and gastrointestinal symptoms. Compared to routine medical care, psychodynamic therapy for IBS and functional dyspepsia improves bowel dysfunction, abdominal pain, and psychological symptoms after one year. However, the supporting studies are methodologically flawed.

One large study demonstrated that brief psychodynamic therapy is acceptable and cost-effective for patients with IBS who have not responded to routine treatments. Psychodynamic interpersonal therapy and paroxetine each improves health-related quality of life but not pain, compared to usual treatment. This improvement cannot be accounted for by improved psychological status. Data from this study suggest that patients with a history of sexual abuse do particularly well.

Hypnotherapy

Hypnotherapy is commonly employed in England and parts of Europe for IBS and functional dyspepsia. The hypnotic state consists of unusual concentration on the suggestion of the therapist and depends upon the willingness of the subject to follow her requests. Following induction, the hypnotherapist uses progressive muscular relaxation with "gut-directed" imagery and suggestions to relax gastrointestinal smooth muscle. A patient is requested to place his hand on his abdomen, to sense a positive feeling of abdominal warmth and increased control over gut function, and to visualize the gut as a gentle flowing river. Patients may practice autohypnosis at home using an audiotape.

Some work shows that hypnotherapy reduces gut contractile activity and increases the pain threshold when a balloon is distended in the rectum, but others fail to confirm this. Other studies show cognitive improvements similar to those following CBT. Controlled trials of hypnotherapy in IBS and functional dyspepsia suggest it is an effective and lasting treatment. It is not known whether hypnotherapy is applicable to patients in primary care. Older patients and those with marked anxiety and atypical symptoms respond less well. As with other psychotherapies, controls for hypnotherapy are difficult to devise and disguise.

Conclusion

This chapter reviews several of the therapies referred to in chapter 16 for treatment of the FGIDs. Despite the admirable efforts of the pharmaceutical industry to develop sophisticated randomized trials for the FGIDs, much more work is required to provide the medical evidence necessary for the rational use of drugs and other treatments. Because there are no cures, the general measures outlined in chapters 13 and 14 are very important, while the more specific agents discussed here are directed against the principal symptoms.

The difficulty in providing controls for FGID psychotherapy trials hampers progress. Psychological difficulties are ubiquitous and their important role in functional disorders should be acknowledged. More severely affected patients are unresponsive to other measures, unable to cope with the symptoms, and suffer from anxiety or depression. They may need psychoactive medication or referral to a mental health professional. In such patients, CBT, hypnotherapy and other psychotherapeutic approaches have much to offer.

Sources

Behar J, Corazziari E, Guelrud M, Hogan WJ, Sherman S, Toouli J. Functional gallbladder and sphincter of Oddi disorders. In: Drossman DA, Corazziari E, Delvaux M, Spiller RC, Talley NJ, Thompson WG, Whitehead WE, eds. *Rome III: The Functional Gastrointestinal Disorders*. McLean, VA: Degnon Associates, Inc.; 2006: 595-635.

Camilleri M, Bueno L, De Ponti F, Fioramonte J, Lydiard RB, Tack J. Pharmacological and pharmacokinetic aspects of functional gastrointestinal disorders. In: Drossman DA, Corazziari E, Delvaux M, Spiller RC, Talley NJ, Thompson WG, Whitehead WE, eds. *Rome III: The Functional Gastrointestinal Disorders*. McLean, VA: Degnon Associates, Inc.: 2006:161-229.

Clouse RE, Mayer EA, Aziz Q, Drossman DA, Dumitrascu DL, Mönnikes H, Naliboff BD. Functional abdominal pain syndrome. In: Drossman DA, Corazziari E, Delvaux M, Spiller RC, Talley NJ, Thompson WG, Whitehead WE, eds. *Rome III:*

The Functional Gastrointestinal Disorders. McLean, VA: Degnon Associates, Inc.; 2006: 557-493.

Creed F, Levy RL, Bradley LA, Drossman DA, Francisconi C, Naliboff BD, Olden KW. Psychosocial aspects of the functional gastrointestinal disorders. In: Drossman DA, Corazziari E, Delvaux M, Spiller RC, Talley NJ, Thompson WG, Whitehead WE, eds. *Rome III: The Functional Gastrointestinal Disorders.* McLean, VA: Degnon Associates, Inc.; 2006:295-267.

Drossman DA, Toner BB, Whitehead WE, Diamant NE, Dalton CB, Duncan S, Emmott S, et al. Cognitive-behavioral therapy versus education and desipramine versus placebo for moderate to severe functional bowel disorders. *Gastroenterology.* 2003;125:19-31.

Galmiche JP, Clouse RE, Bálint A, Cook IJ, Kahrilas PJ, Paterson WG, Smout AJPM. Functional esophageal disorders. In: Drossman DA, Corazziari E, Delvaux M, Spiller RC, Talley NJ, Thompson WG, Whitehead W, eds. *Rome III: The Functional Gastrointestinal Disorders.* McLean, VA: Degnon Associates, Inc.; 2006:369-417.

Klein KB. Controlled treatment trials in the irritable bowel syndrome: a critique. *Gastroenterology.* 1988; 95:232-241.

Longstreth GF, Thompson WG, Chey WD, Houghton LA, Mearin F, Spiller RC. Functional bowel disorders. In: Drossman DA, Corazziari E, Delvaux M, Spiller RC, Talley NJ, Thompson WG, Whitehead WE, eds. *Rome III: The Functional Gastrointestinal Disorders.* McLean, VA: Degnon Associates, Inc.; 2006:487-555.

Spiller R. Clinical update: irritable bowel syndrome. *Lancet.* 2007;369(9573): 1586-1588.

Tack J, Talley NJ, Camilleri M, Holtmann G, Hu P, Malagalada J-R, Stanghellini V. Functional gastroduodenal disorders. In: Drossman DA, Corazziari E, Delvaux M, Spiller RC, Talley NJ, Thompson WG, Whitehead WE, editors. *Rome III: The Functional Gastrointestinal Disorders.* McLean, VA: Degnon Associates, Inc.; 2006: 419-485

Thompson WG. *The Ulcer Story: The Authoritative Guide to Ulcers, Dyspepsia, and Heartburn.* New York: Plenum Publishing; 1996.

Thompson WG. Review article: the treatment of irritable bowel syndrome. *Aliment Pharmacol Therap.* 2002;16:1395-1406.

Thompson WG, Heaton KW. *Fast Facts: Irritable Bowel Syndrome*, 2nd ed. Oxford: Health Press; 2003.

Wald A, Bharucha AE, Enck P, Rao S. Functional anorectal disorders. In: Drossman DA, Corazziari E, Delvaux M, Spiller RC, Talley NJ, Thompson WG, Whitehead WE, eds. *Rome III: The Functional Gastrointestinal Disorders.* McLean, VA: Degnon Associates, Inc.; 2006:639-685.

Whorwell PJ, Altringer L, Morel J, Bond Y, Charbonneau D, O'Mahony L, Kiely B, Shanahan F, Qugley EM. Efficacy of an encapsulated probiotic Bifidobacterium infantis 35624 in women with irritable bowel syndrome. *Am J Gastroenterol.* 2006;101(7):1581-1590.

EPILOGUE
The Challenges

Introduction

These pages summarize a remarkable progress in our understanding of the functional gastrointestinal disorders (FGIDs). Figure F-1 illustrates the increase in annual scientific reports of only one FGID, the irritable bowel syndrome (IBS), since the Rome process began. The Rome classification enables clinical studies that are applicable to individual patients. Doctors can diagnose these disorders with confidence, and without costly and fruitless testing. No longer are people with functional complaints stigmatized as lacking a real disease. We have learned that functional gut symptoms are very common in the community, and when they are severe they can be costly and associated with psychological and somatic comorbidities that collectively impair a person's quality of life. While the nature of these disorders puzzles us still, we are beginning to see that medical evidence supports the efficacy of some treatments.

Where to now? The fundamental debate remains. Will we find a concrete explanation for each disorder as research closes in on the gut and its enteric and central controllers, or will each person's symptoms prove to have many causes—perhaps an etiology as unique as his fingerprint or his personality? Neither view contradicts the biopsychosocial nature of individual patients, but the pursuit of specific causes will continue to challenge us. Each working team responsible for a chapter in *Rome III: The Functional Gastrointestinal Disorders* proposes future scientific initiatives. These glimpse the future of FGID research—the collective vision of eighty-seven experts from around the world. They are wish lists to be sure, but together they express the vastness and complexity of the challenges to all who are interested in improving the lives of those with functional gut disorders. To this writer the challenges implied by these initiatives can be grouped in three categories: the solitudes, the loci of research, and the promotion of the therapeutic relationship.

The Solitudes

While basic scientists urge that more resources be deployed for the understanding of gut function and dysfunction at a molecular level, patients and clinicians seek better application of current knowledge to the amelioration of symptoms at a human level. Each group constitutes a solitude that operates in its own sphere, only marginally aware of the others. Rather than complement each other, the solitudes sometimes conflict. The scientist sees a gap in understanding and places little value in the anecdote, the diagnosis, or the complexity of clinical practice. The proposition must be proven or it doesn't exist. Clinicians and patients, impatient with the slow progress of research, must daily confront the fuzzy face of illness. Their decisions are based on experience and the results of their doctor/patient interactions—each in turn so different from one another that the application of science seems problematic. The scientist looks at the FGIDs and seeks to explain them. Hence the illness is defined by a physiological phenomenon or not at all. The problem for practicing doctors is that "not at all" defines most of their patients. They cannot wait for science. For some scientists, the *Rome* criteria may be "castles in the sky," but for clinical researchers, doctors, and patients they offer an opportunity to replace confusion with order.

Many gastroenterologists claim that patients with the FGIDs constitute over half their practices and that they struggle to meet their needs. General practitioners and family doctors may see only one or two cases a week and, knowing the patient's family and personality, do not usually consider the disorders a great problem compared to the rest of their daily work. They send their difficult cases on. Mental health professionals see the FGIDs through a psychological prism, since FGID patients without psychopathology will not be referred to them. Each medical specialty has its own solitude—its own world view of the functional disorders. Finally we cannot, must not, forget the ultimate solitude—that of the patient.

The first great challenge then is to bring the solitudes together. For even the most empirical of scientists must be familiar with the problems that patients and clinicians confront so that they have relevant scientific issues to address. Conversely, even the most pragmatic physicians and patients need help in deciding how best to apply existing knowledge to illness. Specialists need to understand that they do not see the universe of those with FGIDs. Indeed, neither do primary care doctors, since most people with such symptoms do not consult doctors.

The Loci of Research

Basic research is important for its own sake. Like art, creative science depends upon the imagination, and there must be a cadre of basic scientists free to explore their ideas. As they work, they sometimes achieve surprising and unintended results that benefit patients far removed from their fields of interest. Good ideas come to the prepared mind. Nevertheless, with the FGIDs much "me-too" research is conducted. For more than a half century, scientists have tried to understand the movements of the gastrointestinal tract in health and disease. Although such work remains important, it cries out for new methods. The Rome basic science and pharmacology committees' suggestions for study of the cellular and neural mechanisms underlying gut functions are more promising. We have learned much about serotonin in the gut, which has resulted in some useful drugs. Surely it is time to study with equal vigor the many other neurotransmitters that inhabit the enteric nervous system. "Visceral hypersensitivity" is a challenging hypothesis, but why is it so seldom demonstrable in individual patients. Are not new paradigms required? Clinical scientists have tabulated the characteristics and prevalences of the disorders in the community, but we know little about their behavior in real-life clinical situations. Armchair academics adopt as their métier meta-analysis and systematic reviews, but existing FGID treatment trials do not justify their subjection to a single analysis. There is an unhealthy concentration of RCTs of new pharmaceuticals, while the use of older drugs and other treatments continues with no supporting evidence. So much FGID data emanates from academe and industry and so little from the frontlines of clinical practice.

The Promotion of the Therapeutic Relationship

The *Rome III* project and this book emphasize the importance of the doctor/patient relationship in the treatment of the FGIDs. Diagnosis, education, reassurance, and empathy can achieve much, especially for illnesses that have no known causes and many influences, and for whose treatment there is no magic bullet. These admirable principles are the life blood of the art and science of medicine, but are often sacrificed for lack of time. Talking to patients is the least rewarded of a doctor's tasks, yet it is the most difficult to do well. Expensive technological procedures such as endoscopy trump face time with patients. Primary care doctors must respond to demands for efficiency by seeing more patients and shortening their visits. Managers who consider such developments to be economical should think again. Data show that FGID patients who are given short shrift by their doctors are more likely to receive inappropriate treatment, to be dissatisfied, to consult again, and to have unsatisfactory outcomes. Is it more economical in time and money to do an endoscopy or remove a gallbladder than to take the time to ensure they are needed?

What to Do?

Solitudes are only broken by communication. Joint meetings of professionals in various fields do bring basic, psychological, and clinical scientists together where they participate in the same agenda. The intent is admirable, but the reality is that the herd instinct of like professionals is strong—the solitudes speak among themselves. Not only are their contributions directed to their own kind, but the program usually permits scientists to leave when their pieces are done and before clinicians who are just arriving present their material. Surely the solution is interdisciplinary interaction. Scientific programs should include workshops and symposia that involve all relevant disciplines and explore opportunities for collaboration. Even the authors of the *Rome* chapters could do more to teach one another. Moreover, with disorders as ubiquitous as the FGIDs, no conference should omit the primary care doctor, upon whose shoulders the responsibility for most patients must fall. Patients could participate as well, keeping in mind that they too have solitudes, and no one person can embody everyone's perspective.

Basic researchers should be free to pursue their imaginations, for it is from them that major advances will come. They need encouragement and funding, of course. However, there should be more diversity in research. There is much more to the enteric nervous system than serotonin, and we know that parts of the brain light up with rectal distension. What is needed are more experiments that address other neurotransmitters and the meaning of that brain activity. To match the financial clout of the pharmaceutical RCT, nongovernment organizations and governments should fund clinical trials of older drugs, diets, and alternative treatments. The literature is littered with dubious small trials executed with poor methodology and few resources. Their systematic review cannot sanitize their poor science. New research initiatives are needed. Funding authorities ought to give priority to unique ideas. Marshall and Warren thought outside the ulcer 'box,' which was obsessed with gastric acid. They studied previously ignored organisms in the stomach, and won the Nobel Prize. No funding agency helped their efforts. We need a cadre of independent FGID researchers beholden neither to industry nor funding orthodoxy who can inject new ideas into FGID research.

In the clinical arena, as an ideal principle of care the family doctor should be in charge. Specialists and psychologists are part of the team, but the generalist who knows the patient, his family, and his comorbidities is best positioned for the patient's long-term care. The family doctor's central role must be supported by functional gut research in primary care.

The most valuable physician resource is time. Doctors need the resolve and incentives to spend more time talking to their patients. When properly conducted, the medical interview should result in a positive doctor/patient relationship, a diagnosis, an educated and reassured patient, a placebo effect, and an evidence-based plan of investigation and management. Doctors and patients should convince those responsible for health care management that this approach not only promotes better care, but also can save money through a satisfied patient and the wise choice of tests and therapy. Satisfied patients who can manage their FGIDs on their own are unlikely to seek further care. Waiting lists would shorten if those not requiring the procedure were not on them.

Education is the key. The solitudes need to educate each other and collectively we need to educate patients, doctors, the public, and health care managers. The Rome Foundation plans a leading role. Through meetings leading up to *Rome IV*, experts will again be convened and interdisciplinary views will be exchanged. Meanwhile, Rome-sponsored working teams address new research issues and resolve old controversies, and the Rome Foundation's competitive grants encourage novel research. Symposia and teaching materials educate professional colleagues and researchers. Perhaps the Foundation should do more to promote the therapeutic relationship. There is much to do.

Conclusion

The Rome process gives us an FGID vocabulary. We now discuss these disorders and know their meaning. Moreover, the Rome classification gives the disorders status as real illnesses, of which no one need be ashamed, and no doctor can shrug off as "all in the head." Using this new vocabulary we have learned who and how many people have the disorders, their demography, their psychosocial characteristics, their associated illnesses, and their health-care-seeking behavior. We are developing the tools to discover their disordered physiology, and to test the usefulness of their putative treatments. Now, we must move on to integrate the disciplines that are investigating and managing these disorders, and direct research into new areas—especially the neurobiology of the gut and the validation of those long-used procedures and treatments that have never been subjected to a modern clinical trial. Most immediately, and perhaps most importantly, we need to convince everyone of the value of the doctor/patient relationship and the time it requires. A five-minute interview may save some money in the short term, but the downstream downsides of an unsatisfied patient who is dismissed with a pill and an unneeded test requisition are substantial.

APPENDIX A
The *Rome III* Diagnostic Criteria for the Functional Gastrointestinal Disorders

The *Rome* criteria for the diagnoses of the functional gastrointestinal disorders (FGIDs) were developed by teams of experts to define patients for scientific study and to help practicing doctors more precisely identify the disorders. They are included here as a convenient reference. The FGIDs that affect adults are described in detail in part 2 of this book. For completeness, the diagnostic criteria for childhood FGIDs are included in this appendix. Apart from listing their diagnostic criteria here, however, *Understanding the Irritable Gut* does not discuss the infant/toddler and child/adolescent disorders

The criteria are not meant for self-diagnosis. A confident diagnosis can only be safely arrived at after a careful history and physical examination by a doctor as described in chapter 5.

As new information becomes available the criteria require updating; the *Rome IV* iteration is planned for 2012. The process is ongoing.

ROME III DIAGNOSTIC CRITERIA FOR ADULTS

A. FUNCTIONAL ESOPHAGEAL DISORDERS

A1. Functional Heartburn
Diagnostic criteria* must include **all** of the following:
1. Burning retrosternal discomfort or pain
2. Absence of evidence that gastroesophageal acid reflux is the cause of the symptom
3. Absence of histopathology-based esophageal motility disorders

* Criteria fulfilled for the last three months with symptom onset at least six months prior to diagnosis

A2. Functional Chest Pain of Presumed Esophageal Origin
Diagnostic criteria* must include **all** of the following:
1. Midline chest pain or discomfort that is not of burning quality
2. Absence of evidence that gastroesophageal reflux is the cause of the symptom
3. Absence of histopathology-based esophageal motility disorders

* Criteria fulfilled for the last three months with symptom onset at least six months prior to diagnosis

A3. Functional Dysphagia
Diagnostic criteria* must include **all** of the following:
1. Sense of solid and/or liquid foods sticking, lodging, or passing abnormally through the esophagus
2. Absence of evidence that gastroesophageal reflux is the cause of the symptom
3. Absence of histopathology-based esophageal motility disorders

* Criteria fulfilled for the last three months with symptom onset at least six months prior to diagnosis

A4. Globus
Diagnostic criteria* must include **all** of the following:
1. Persistent or intermittent, nonpainful sensation of a lump or foreign body in the throat
2. Occurrence of the sensation between meals
3. Absence of dysphagia or odynophagia
4. Absence of evidence that gastroesophageal reflux is the cause of the symptom
5. Absence of histopathology-based esophageal motility disorders

* Criteria fulfilled for the last three months with symptom onset at least six months prior to diagnosis

B. FUNCTIONAL GASTRODUODENAL DISORDERS

B1. Functional Dyspepsia
Diagnostic criteria* must include
1. One or more of the following:
    a. Bothersome postprandial fullness
    b. Early satiation
    c. Epigastric pain
    d. Epigastric burning
AND
2. No evidence of structural disease (including at upper endoscopy) that is likely to explain the symptoms

* Criteria fulfilled for the last three months with symptom onset at least six months prior to diagnosis

B1a. *Postprandial Distress Syndrome*
Diagnostic criteria* must include **one or both** of the following:
1. Bothersome postprandial fullness, occurring after ordinary-sized meals, at least several times per week
2. Early satiation that prevents finishing a regular meal, at least several times per week

* Criteria fulfilled for the last three months with symptom onset at least six months prior to diagnosis

Supportive criteria
1. Upper abdominal bloating or postprandial nausea or excessive belching can be present.
2. Epigastric pain syndrome may coexist.

B1b. Epigastric Pain Syndrome
Diagnostic criteria* must include **all** of the following:

1. Pain or burning localized to the epigastrium of at least moderate severity, at least once per week
2. Pain is intermittent
3. Pain is not generalized or localized to other abdominal or chest regions
4. Pain is not relieved by defecation or passage of flatus
5. Symptoms do not fulfill criteria for gallbladder and sphincter of Oddi disorders

* Criteria fulfilled for the last three months with symptom onset at least six months prior to diagnosis

Supportive criteria

1. The pain may be of a burning quality, but without a retrosternal component.
2. The pain is commonly induced or relieved by ingestion of a meal, but may occur while fasting.
3. Postprandial distress syndrome may coexist.

B2. Belching Disorders

B2a. Aerophagia
Diagnostic criteria* must include **all** of the following:

1. Troublesome repetitive belching at least several times a week
2. Air swallowing that is objectively observed or measured

* Criteria fulfilled for the last three months with symptom onset at least six months prior to diagnosis

B2b. Unspecified Excessive Belching
Diagnostic criteria* must include **all** of the following:

1. Troublesome repetitive belching at least several times a week
2. No evidence that excessive air swallowing underlies the symptom

* Criteria fulfilled for the last three months with symptom onset at least six months prior to diagnosis

B3. Nausea and Vomiting Disorders

B3a. Chronic Idiopathic Nausea
Diagnostic criteria* must include **all** of the following:
1. Bothersome nausea occurring at least several times per week
2. Nausea not usually associated with vomiting
3. Absence of abnormalities at upper endoscopy or metabolic disease that explains the nausea

* Criteria fulfilled for the last three months with symptom onset at least six months prior to diagnosis

B3b. Functional Vomiting
Diagnostic criteria* must include **all** of the following:
1. On average one or more episodes of vomiting per week
2. Absence of criteria for an eating disorder, rumination, or major psychiatric disease according to the *Diagnostic and Statistical Manual of Mental Disorders IV* (DSM-IV)
3. Absence of self-induced vomiting and chronic cannabinoid use and absence of abnormalities in the central nervous system or metabolic diseases to explain the recurrent vomiting

* Criteria fulfilled for the last three months with symptom onset at least six months prior to diagnosis

B3c. Cyclic Vomiting Syndrome
Diagnostic criteria must include **all** of the following:
1. Stereotypical episodes of vomiting regarding onset (acute) and duration (less than one week)
2. Three or more discrete episodes in the prior year
3. Absence of nausea and vomiting between episodes

Supportive criterion

History or family history of migraine headaches

B4. Rumination Syndrome in Adults
Diagnostic criteria must include **both** of the following:
1. Persistent or recurrent regurgitation of recently ingested food into the mouth with subsequent spitting or remastication and swallowing
2. Regurgitation not preceded by retching

Supportive criteria
1. Regurgitation events are usually not preceded by nausea.
2. Process ceases when the regurgitated material becomes acidic.
3. Regurgitant contains recognizable food with a pleasant taste.

C. FUNCTIONAL BOWEL DISORDERS

C1. Irritable Bowel Syndrome
*Diagnostic criteria**
Recurrent abdominal pain or discomfort** at least three days per month in the last six months associated with **two or more** of the following:
1. Improvement with defecation
2. Onset associated with a change in frequency of stool
3. Onset associated with a change in form (appearance) of stool

* Criteria fulfilled for the last three months with symptom onset at least six months prior to diagnosis

** "Discomfort" means an uncomfortable sensation not described as pain. In pathophysiology research and clinical trials, a pain/discomfort frequency of at least two days a week during screening evaluation is recommended for subject eligibility.

C2. Functional Bloating
Diagnostic criteria* must include **both** of the following:
1. Recurrent feeling of bloating or visible distension at least three days per month in the last three months
2. Insufficient criteria for a diagnosis of functional dyspepsia, irritable bowel syndrome, or other functional GI disorder

* Criteria fulfilled for the last three months with symptom onset at least six months prior to diagnosis

C3. Functional Constipation
Diagnostic criteria* must include **two or more** of the following:
1. Straining during at least 25% of defecations
2. Lumpy or hard stools in at least 25% of defecations
3. Sensation of incomplete evacuation for at least 25% of defecations
4. Sensation of anorectal obstruction/blockage for at least 25% of defecations
5. Manual maneuvers to facilitate at least 25% of defecations (e.g., digital evacuation, support of the pelvic floor)
6. Fewer than three defecations per week
7. Loose stools are rarely present without the use of laxatives
8. Insufficient criteria for irritable bowel syndrome

* Criteria fulfilled for the last three months with symptom onset at least six months prior to diagnosis

C4. Functional Diarrhea
*Diagnostic criterion**
Loose (mushy) or watery stools without pain occurring in at least 75% of stools
* Criterion fulfilled for the last three months with symptom onset at least six months prior to diagnosis

C5. Unspecified Functional Bowel Disorder
*Diagnostic criterion**
Bowel symptoms not attributable to an organic etiology that do not meet criteria for the previously defined categories
* Criterion fulfilled for the last three months with symptom onset at least six months prior to diagnosis

D. FUNCTIONAL ABDOMINAL PAIN SYNDROME

D. Functional Abdominal Pain Syndrome

Diagnostic criteria* must include **all** of the following:

1. Continuous or nearly continuous abdominal pain
2. No or only occasional relationship of pain with physiological events (e.g., eating, defecation, or menses)
3. Some loss of daily functioning
4. No feigning of pain (e.g., malingering)
5. Insufficient symptoms to meet criteria for another functional gastrointestinal disorder that would explain the pain

* Criteria fulfilled for the last three months with symptom onset at least six months prior to diagnosis

E. FUNCTIONAL GALLBLADDER AND SPHINCTER OF ODDI DISORDERS

Diagnostic criteria must include episodes of pain located in the epigastrium and/or right upper quadrant and **all** of the following:

1. Episodes lasting thirty minutes or longer
2. Recurrent symptoms occurring at different intervals (not daily)
3. Pain building up to a steady level
4. Pain moderate-to-severe enough to interrupt the patient's daily activities or lead to an emergency department visit
5. Pain not relieved by bowel movements
6. Pain not relieved by postural change
7. Pain not relieved by antacids
8. Exclusion of other structural disease that would explain the symptoms

Supportive criteria

The pain may present with one or more of the following characteristics:

1. Associated nausea and vomiting
2. Radiates to the back and/or right infrasubscapular region
3. Awakens the patient from sleep in the middle of the night

E1. Functional Gallbladder Disorder

Diagnostic criteria must include **all** of the following:

1. Criteria for functional gallbladder and sphincter of Oddi disorders
2. Gallbladder is present
3. Normal liver enzymes, conjugated bilirubin, and amylase/lipase

E2. Functional Biliary Sphincter of Oddi Disorder
Diagnostic criteria must include **both** of the following:
1. Criteria for functional gallbladder and sphincter of Oddi disorders
2. Normal amylase/lipase

Supportive criterion

Elevated serum transaminases, alkaline phosphatase, or conjugated bilirubin temporarily related to at least two pain episodes

E3. Functional Pancreatic Sphincter of Oddi Disorder
Diagnostic criteria must include **both** of the following:
1. Criteria for functional gallbladder and sphincter of Oddi disorders
2. Elevated amylase/lipase

F. FUNCTIONAL ANORECTAL DISORDERS

F1. Functional Fecal Incontinence
Diagnostic criteria*
1. Recurrent uncontrolled passage of fecal material in an individual with a developmental age of at least four years and one or more of the following:
    a. Abnormal functioning of normally innervated and structurally intact muscles
    b. Minor abnormalities of sphincter structure and/or innervation
    c. Normal or disordered bowel habits (i.e., fecal retention or diarrhea)
    d. Psychological causes

AND

2. Exclusion of **all** the following:
    a. Abnormal innervation caused by lesion(s) within the brain (e.g., dementia), spinal cord, or sacral nerve roots, or mixed lesions (e.g., multiple sclerosis), or as part of a generalized peripheral or autonomic neuropathy (e.g., due to diabetes)
    b. Anal sphincter abnormalities associated with a multisystem disease (e.g., scleroderma)
    c. Structural or neurogenic abnormalities believed to be the major or primary cause of fecal incontinence

* Criteria fulfilled for the last three months

F2. Functional Anorectal Pain

F2a. Chronic Proctalgia
Diagnostic criteria* must include **all** of the following:
1. Chronic or recurrent rectal pain or aching
2. Episodes last twenty minutes or longer
3. Exclusion of other causes of rectal pain such as ischemia, inflammatory bowel disease, cryptitis, intramuscular abscess, anal fissure, hemorrhoids, prostatitis, and coccygodynia

* Criteria fulfilled for the last three months with symptom onset at least six months prior to diagnosis

Chronic proctalgia may be further characterized into levator ani syndrome or unspecified anorectal pain based on digital rectal examination.

F2a.1. Levator Ani Syndrome
Diagnostic criterion
Symptom criteria for chronic proctalgia and tenderness during posterior traction on the puborectalis

F2a.2. Unspecified Functional Anorectal Pain
Diagnostic criterion
Symptom criteria for chronic proctalgia but no tenderness during posterior traction on the puborectalis

F2b. Proctalgia Fugax
Diagnostic criteria* must include **all** of the following:
1. Recurrent episodes of pain localized to the anus or lower rectum
2. Episodes lasting from seconds to minutes
3. No anorectal pain between episodes

* For research purposes criteria must be fulfilled for three months; however, clinical diagnosis and evaluation may be made prior to three months.

F3. Functional Defecation Disorders
Diagnostic criteria*
1. Satisfies diagnostic criteria for functional constipation**
2. During repeated attempts to defecate, must have **at least two** of the following:
    a. Evidence of impaired evacuation, based on balloon expulsion test or imaging
    b. Inappropriate contraction of the pelvic floor muscles (i.e., anal sphincter or puborectalis) or less than 20% relaxation of basal resting sphincter pressure by manometry, imaging, or electromyograph (EMG)
    c. Inadequate propulsive forces assessed by manometry or imaging

* Criteria fulfilled for the last three months with symptom onset at least six months prior to diagnosis

** Diagnostic criteria for functional constipation:
(1) Must include **two or more** of the following:
    (a) Straining during at least 25% of defecations
    (b) Lumpy or hard stools in at least 25% of defecations
    (c) Sensation of incomplete evacuation for at least 25% of defecations
    (d) Sensation of anorectal obstruction/blockage for at least 25% of defecations
    (e) Manual maneuvers to facilitate at least 25% of defecations (e.g., digital evacuation, support of the pelvic floor)
    (f) Fewer than three defecations per week
(2) Loose stools are rarely present without the use of laxatives.
(3) Insufficient criteria for irritable bowel syndrome.

F3a. Dyssynergic Defecation
Diagnostic criterion
Inappropriate contraction of the pelvic floor or less than 20% relaxation of basal resting sphincter pressure with adequate propulsive forces during attempted defecation

F3b. Inadequate Defecatory Propulsion
Diagnostic criterion
Inadequate propulsive forces with or without inappropriate contraction or less than 20% relaxation of the anal sphincter during attempted defecation

ROME III DIAGNOSTIC CRITERIA FOR CHILDREN AND ADOLESCENTS

G. CHILDHOOD FUNCTIONAL GI DISORDERS: INFANT/TODDLER

G1. Infant Regurgitation
Diagnostic criteria must include **both** of the following in otherwise healthy infants three weeks to twelve months of age:
1. Regurgitation two or more times per day for three or more weeks
2. No retching, hematemesis, aspiration, apnea, failure to thrive, feeding or swallowing difficulties, or abnormal posturing

G2. Infant Rumination Syndrome
Diagnostic criteria must include **all** of the following for at least three months:
1. Repetitive contractions of the abdominal muscles, diaphragm, and tongue
2. Regurgitation of gastric content into the mouth, which is either expectorated or rechewed and reswallowed
3. Three or more of the following:
   a. Onset between three and eight months
   b. Does not respond to management for gastroesophageal reflux disease, or to anticholinergic drugs, hand restraints, formula changes, and gavage or gastrostomy feedings
   c. Unaccompanied by signs of nausea or distress
   d. Does not occur during sleep and when the infant is interacting with individuals in the environment

G3. Cyclic Vomiting Syndrome
Diagnostic criteria must include **both** of the following:
1. Two or more periods of intense nausea and unremitting vomiting or retching lasting hours to days
2. Return to usual state of health lasting weeks to months

Note: The diagnostic criteria for pediatric FGIDs are included here for completeness. The pediatric disorders are not discussed in this book.

G4. Infant Colic

Diagnostic criteria must include **all** of the following in infants from birth to four months of age:

1. Paroxysms of irritability, fussing, or crying that start and stop without obvious cause
2. Episodes lasting three or more hours per day and occurring at least three days per week for at least one week
3. No failure to thrive

G5. Functional Diarrhea

Diagnostic criteria must include **all** of the following:

1. Daily painless, recurrent passage of three or more large, unformed stools
2. Symptoms that last more than four weeks
3. Onset of symptoms that begins between six and thirty-six months of age
4. Passage of stools that occurs during waking hours
5. There is no failure to thrive if caloric intake is adequate

G6. Infant Dyschezia

Diagnostic criteria must include **both** of the following in an infant less than six months of age:

1. At least ten minutes of straining and crying before successful passage of soft stools
2. No other health problems

G7. Functional Constipation

Diagnostic criteria must include one month of **at least two** of the following in infants up to four years of age:

1. Two or fewer defecations per week
2. At least one episode per week of incontinence after the acquisition of toileting skills
3. History of excessive stool retention
4. History of painful or hard bowel movements
5. Presence of a large fecal mass in the rectum
6. History of large-diameter stools that may obstruct the toilet

Accompanying symptoms may include irritability, decreased appetite, and/or early satiety. The accompanying symptoms disappear immediately following passage of a large stool.

Note: The diagnostic criteria for pediatric FGIDs are included here for completeness. The pediatric disorders are not discussed in this book.

H. CHILDHOOD FUNCTIONAL GI DISORDERS: CHILD/ADOLESCENT

H1. Vomiting and Aerophagia

H1a. Adolescent Rumination Syndrome
Diagnostic criteria* must include **all** of the following:
1. Repeated painless regurgitation and rechewing or expulsion of food that
   a. begin soon after ingestion of a meal
   b. do not occur during sleep
   c. do not respond to standard treatment for gastroesophageal reflux
2. No retching
3. No evidence of an inflammatory, anatomic, metabolic, or neoplastic process that explains the subject's symptoms

* Criteria fulfilled for the last three months with symptom onset at least six months prior to diagnosis

H1b. Cyclic Vomiting Syndrome (CVS)
Diagnostic criteria must include **both** of the following:
1. Two or more periods of intense nausea and unremitting vomiting or retching lasting hours to days
2. Return to usual state of health lasting weeks to months

H1c. Aerophagia
Diagnostic criteria* must include **at least two** of the following:
1. Air swallowing
2. Abdominal distention due to intraluminal air
3. Repetitive belching and/or increased flatus

* Criteria fulfilled at least once per week for at least two months prior to diagnosis

---

Note: The diagnostic criteria for pediatric FGIDs are included here for completeness. The pediatric disorders are not discussed in this book.

H2. Abdominal Pain-Related Functional GI Disorders

H2a. Functional Dyspepsia
Diagnostic criteria* must include **all** of the following:
1. Persistent or recurrent pain or discomfort centered in the upper abdomen (above the umbilicus)
2. Not relieved by defecation or associated with the onset of a change in stool frequency or stool form (i.e., not irritable bowel syndrome)
3. No evidence of an inflammatory, anatomic, metabolic, or neoplastic process that explains the subject's symptoms

* Criteria fulfilled at least once per week for at least two months prior to diagnosis

H2b. Irritable Bowel Syndrome
Diagnostic criteria* must include **both** of the following:
1. Abdominal discomfort** or pain associated with **two or more** of the following at least 25% of the time:
   a. Improvement with defecation
   b. Onset associated with a change in frequency of stool
   c. Onset associated with a change in form (appearance) of stool
2. No evidence of an inflammatory, anatomic, metabolic, or neoplastic process that explains the subject's symptoms

* Criteria fulfilled at least once per week for at least two months prior to diagnosis

**"Discomfort" means an uncomfortable sensation not described as pain.

Note: The diagnostic criteria for pediatric FGIDs are included here for completeness. The pediatric disorders are not discussed in this book.

H2c. Abdominal Migraine

Diagnostic criteria* must include **all** of the following:

1. Paroxysmal episodes of intense, acute periumbilical pain that lasts for one hour or more
2. Intervening periods of usual health lasting weeks to months
3. The pain interferes with normal activities
4. The pain is associated with two of the following:
   a. Anorexia
   b. Nausea
   c. Vomiting
   d. Headache
   e. Photophobia
   f. Pallor
5. No evidence of an inflammatory, anatomic, metabolic, or neoplastic process considered that explains the subject's symptoms

* Criteria fulfilled two or more times in the preceding twelve months.

H2d. Childhood Functional Abdominal Pain

Diagnostic criteria* must include **all** of the following:

1. Episodic or continuous abdominal pain
2. Insufficient criteria for other FGIDs
3. No evidence of an inflammatory, anatomic, metabolic, or neoplastic process that explains the subject's symptoms

* Criteria fulfilled at least once per week for at least two months prior to diagnosis

H2d1. Childhood Functional Abdominal Pain Syndrome

Diagnostic criteria* must satisfy criteria for childhood functional abdominal pain and have at least 25% of the time **one or more** of the following:

1. Some of loss of daily functioning
2. Additional somatic symptoms such as headache, limb pain, or difficulty sleeping

*Criteria fulfilled at least once per week for at least two months prior to diagnosis

---

Note: The diagnostic criteria for pediatric FGIDs are included here for completeness. The pediatric disorders are not discussed in this book.

H3. Constipation and Incontinence

H3a. Functional Constipation
Diagnostic criteria* must include **two or more** of the following in a child with a developmental age of at least four years with insufficient criteria for diagnosis of IBS:

1. Two or fewer defecations in the toilet per week
2. At least one episode of fecal incontinence per week
3. History of retentive posturing or excessive volitional stool retention
4. History of painful or hard bowel movements
5. Presence of a large fecal mass in the rectum
6. History of large-diameter stools that may obstruct the toilet

*Criteria fulfilled at least once per week for at least two months prior to diagnosis

H3b. Nonretentive Fecal Incontinence
Diagnostic criteria* must include **all** of the following in a child with a developmental age at least four years:

1. Defecation into places inappropriate to the social context at least once per month
2. No evidence of an inflammatory, anatomic, metabolic, or neoplastic process that explains the subject's symptoms
3. No evidence of fecal retention

*Criteria fulfilled for at least two months prior to diagnosis

---

Note: The diagnostic criteria for pediatric FGIDs are included here for completeness. The pediatric disorders are not discussed in this book.

APPENDIX B
Some Tests Commonly Used in the Investigation of the Functional Gastrointestinal Disorders

This appendix briefly describes some of the investigations mentioned in the preceding chapters. The manner in which these procedures are conducted differs from center to center, although the principles are similar. For more information, readers should refer to standard medical texts or to a local procedural protocol.

Endoscopy

Endoscopy is usually performed by a gastroenterologist or surgeon in an authorized facility with specially trained endoscopy staff. The facility must be equipped with equipment suitable for cardiac or respiratory emergencies. Endoscopy employs a tube-like device that is passed through the mouth or anus through which the examiner can see the gastrointestinal tract. Modern instruments have minute cameras on their tips that project the image onto a video screen. Endoscopes are equipped with ports or passages through which air and water can be passed and excess fluids can be sucked back. Biopsy forceps, polyp snares, and other instruments can pass through these ports as well. An external lamp emits light that is transmitted through the instrument into the intestinal tract. Such instruments can be designed for examination of the upper gastrointestinal tract, the sigmoid colon, the colon, the small intestines, and the biliary tree.

Upper gastrointestinal endoscopy refers to the examination of the upper gastrointestinal tract: the esophagus, stomach, and duodenum. It is known as *esophagogastroduodenoscopy (EGD)*, and is indicated when there are unexplained upper gastrointestinal symptoms that are unresponsive to diet or drugs. The most common indications are dyspepsia (upper abdominal pain or discomfort), persistent heartburn, bleeding from the upper gut, and anemia. Less common reasons for the test are an abnormal upper-gut x-ray, difficulty swallowing, unexplained weight loss, or suspicion or strong family history of esophageal or gastric cancer. The most common findings are a gastric or duodenal ulcer or esophagitis (inflammation of the esophagus). More commonly still, there are no findings—which is normally the case in the FGIDs, notably functional dyspepsia.

The stomach must be empty for the procedure, so a patient must fast from midnight the night before. If the test is scheduled for later in the day, a light breakfast may be consumed. To begin, the endoscopist or the endoscopy nurse applies a topical anesthetic spray or gel to the patient's throat to suppress the gag reflex.

Normally, the patient lies on the left side on an examining table. A mouthpiece is placed between the teeth to permit passage of the endoscope, which protects both the teeth and the instrument. The endoscope is then passed through the mouthpiece and gently brought up against the throat by the examiner's finger. The patient is urged to swallow the tube. The endoscopist carefully inspects the esophagus, the stomach, and the first part of the duodenum. Regular breathing inhibits gagging and maintains good blood-oxygen saturation. The stomach is usually collapsed, so the examiner will inflate it with air via the endoscope. This may produce a feeling of fullness or discomfort. The gut itself is insensitive, so the test is usually painless, but occasionally it can be uncomfortable. There is a tendency to gag. The procedure usually takes about ten minutes, and any discomfort ceases when the instrument is removed. When the local anesthetic wears off, a transient sore throat is normal.

Endoscopic retrograde cholangeopancreatography uses an endoscope with large channels through which may be passed smaller devices to probe the bile and pancreatic ducts. Ample sedation is required because the procedure can be lengthy. Entry into the ducts is technically difficult and the procedure is monitored by x-ray imaging using a fluoroscope. The procedure can result in serious complications such as pancreatitis, perforation, bleeding, or bile-duct infection.

Enteroscopy is the examination of the small intestine with a longer endoscope that is capable of passing beyond the duodenum into the jejunum. It can be a very lengthy procedure and is uncommonly performed.

Colonoscopy and *sigmoidoscopy*. Colonoscopy is an examination whereby an endoscope is inserted through the anus to inspect the entire colon. Sigmoidoscopy is similar, but reaches only the left side of the colon—up to near the splenic flexure. It can be done with little or no sedation in a doctor's office.

Colonoscopy is indicated for the diagnosis of diseases that cause acute and chronic diarrhea, chronic constipation, intestinal bleeding, and for the early detection and management of colon polyps and cancer. Chronic diarrhea may be due to ulcerative colitis or Crohn's disease, both of which need biopsy confirmation. Bleeding has many causes, but it is important to rule out colon cancer or polyps. Other reasons for the test are unexplained weight loss or a strong family history of cancer. Colon carcinoma is the second most common cancer; many groups advocate a screening sigmoidoscopy or colonoscopy for everyone over fifty years of age. However, the most common cause of colon pain and change in bowel habit is the irritable bowel syndrome, for which no abnormalities are discovered.

For a sigmoidoscopy, the patient must take a phosphate enema (Fleet) about two hours before the test. A light meal is permitted in the hours before the test. For colonoscopy, it is imperative that the entire colon be clean. Only fluids are allowed after noon the day before the procedure. One preparation is the ingestion at noon and evening the day before of 60 ml of a phosphate solution (Oral Fleet). An alternative is the ingestion over the previous twelve-to-eighteen hours of four liters of a polyethylene glycol (PEG) solution (CoLyte, GoLYTELy, Peglyte). These solutions cause a profuse diarrhea that should be clear by the time of the procedure. These preparations may be unpleasant, and sometimes cause nausea and cramps. Nevertheless, they are safe when taken with ample clear fluids, and necessary if the examination is to be optimal. Elderly persons should not be alone when undergoing these preparations.

Normally, the patient lies on the left side on an examining table with knees drawn up. The examiner first examines the anal canal with a gloved finger to check for any local disease and to lubricate the passage. The colonoscope is passed through the anus into the rectum. Although intricate controls help direct the tip of the instrument, advancement depends upon the operator pushing it. Because the colon has many sharp angles, the colonoscope tip frequently abuts on a curve. Sometimes, the sigmoid colon and the splenic and hepatic flexures are especially difficult to pass. The advancing tip stretches the colon, which sometimes causes pain. The doctor and nurse then have a repertoire of maneuvers to help the instrument advance. These include alternately withdrawing and advancing, pressing on the abdomen to lessen the tendency of the tube to bulge, and instructing the patient to assume different positions. The colon is usually collapsed, so the examiner must inflate it through the colonoscope. This may produce a feeling of fullness or discomfort. Colonoscopy permits examination of the entire colon and sometimes the lower small bowel.

Everyone is built a little differently. Sometimes the test proceeds rapidly and painlessly. For others, it is more difficult and sometimes uncomfortable as the instrument stretches the organ. On the other hand, procedures done *through* the colonoscope are painless. The lining of the bowel lacks pain receptors, so biopsies are not felt. Even a large polyp can be removed painlessly.

Precautions

If the patient is diabetic or on medication, diet and pill-taking must be adjusted to account for the fasting period. People taking anticoagulants or aspirin must be advised how to proceed, because bleeding can follow biopsy or removal of a polyp. If possible, aspirin should be stopped a week prior to the procedure.

As with all medical procedures, patients who are undergoing endoscopy must sign a consent form to acknowledge the benefits and risks. Normally, endoscopy is very safe. Bleeding or perforation of the gut occurs rarely, usually when the area being examined is diseased, or when a biopsy or polyp removal is undertaken.

Sedation

For a routine EGD, sedation is often given to reduce the tendency to gag during introduction of the endoscope and to lessen the inevitable anxiety associated with the test. In some centers endoscopy patients receive only local anesthesia to the throat. Usually, sedation is given by intravenous injection immediately prior to the test. For sigmoidoscopy, sedation is seldom necessary. The procedure is uncomfortable—even painful—but usually brief. Colonoscopy requires sedation, which is usually injected through an intravenous line. Patients are not put to sleep because they must be conscious and cooperative ("conscious sedation"). The medications are generally safe and effective, but require a recovery period.

Sedated patients must have someone responsible to take them home. A patient may not remember or fully understand the explanation of the procedure given after the test. Too much sedation (and tolerances differ) risks arrested breathing or aspiration of gastric contents into the lungs (another reason to be fasting!). If sedation is given, a device is clipped to a finger that enables the nurse to monitor the heart rate and blood-oxygen saturation.

Afterwards

If there is no sedation, the doctor can discuss the results of the test and their implications promptly. However, a sedated patient must lie in the recovery area for monitoring until he is fully alert; it is unsafe to drive for 24 hours. In this case, discussion must wait.

A negative test is usually very good news. Although FGID symptoms are sometimes severe, it should be a relief to the patient to know there is no life-threatening disease. Therefore the examiner must explain the meaning of the test results as soon as possible. For a sedated patient, that implies a prompt return visit.

Imaging Procedures
Barium Studies

A long-established method of visualizing the gastrointestinal tract is to inject a concentrated barium paste into the gastrointestinal tract and obtain radiographs (x-rays). Since barium blocks the rays, an outline of the gut appears on the radiograph. If carefully done, tumors, ulcers and other lesions can be discovered in this way. If the barium is swallowed, the procedure is known as a barium swallow, or *barium series*. A *small-bowel enema* requires injection of barium directly into the duodenum through a tube. If the barium is injected into the colon through the anus, it is called a *barium enema*. These barium studies are less commonly performed now that various endoscopic procedures can visualize most of the gut. Barium is sometimes used to assess esophageal function or to study defecation, as in *defecography*.

Abdominal Ultrasound

Ultrasound produces high-frequency sound waves that penetrate the body, casting shadows of body structures on a sensitized film or video. Unlike radiographs, ultrasound does not damage tissue, so the procedure is a safe and important means to examine the abdomen. The patient must be fasting, and the bladder must be full. After positioning the patient on the examining table, a technician moves a lubricated probe about the abdomen to secure the images. This painless procedure can show thickened loops of bowel or detect an abscess. Ultrasound can be used to examine abdominal or liver masses and to detect gallstones. It can identify pancreatitis or pancreatic tumors. It is also used to examine anorectal structures. In patients with FGIDs, the test is usually normal.

Endoscopic Ultrasound

Ultrasound probes placed on endoscopes permit more precise endoscopic examination of areas around the upper gastrointestinal tract. The technique detects and evaluates pancreatic tumors and gallstones in the common bile duct. It can also provide information about the extent of tumor spread in the esophagus, stomach, and proximal jejunum.

Computed Tomography (CT)

This x-ray technology enables cross-sectional views of the body. A CT of the abdomen helps detect complications of peptic ulcer such as perforation, or tumors of the upper gut or liver.

Magnetic Resonance Imaging (MRI)

MRI is a more recent technology that detects various elements in tissues and provides an image without tissue-damaging radiation. Because a strong magnetic field is used, individuals with implanted medical objects cannot undergo this procedure. MRI more clearly separates abnormalities of different densities than other imaging methods do, and can distinguish a fluid collection from a tumor or blood from a cyst. Like CT, it allows both cross-sectional and sagittal views. However, MRI is best with a stationary subject and the the gut is always moving. A variation of MRI known as *functional MRI* is used experimentally in FGID patients to quantify activity in various parts of the brain.

Esophageal Motility

This procedure measures pressures within the esophagus. An assembly of either fluid-perfused catheters connected to transducers, or solid-state sensors is passed into the esophagus of a fasting patient to measure pressures at intervals within the lumen. These are recorded on a monitor and paper tracings of the intraesophageal pressures are obtained. This procedure measures the pace and force of esophageal peristalsis and the pressures exerted by the upper and lower esophageal sphincters when they first relax, and then close, in response to a swallow.

An esophageal motility test is particularly useful in confirming a diagnosis of achalasia where peristalsis is weak or absent and the lower esophageal sphincter fails to relax in response to a swallow. In people with the functional esophageal disorders, and sometimes in normal people, abnormal esophageal contractions may be identified by esophageal manometry. So far, researchers have been unable to relate these phenomena to symptoms, and their significance is unknown.

Ambulatory Twenty-four-hour pH Monitoring

Sometimes it unclear whether chest pain, heartburn, or other chest sensation is due to gastroesophageal reflux. Because it is difficult to monitor daily and nocturnal symptoms in a clinic, an indwelling apparatus may be used to record the pH of the lower esophagus while the patient goes about his or her daily activities over a twenty-four-hour period. Using an "event button," the patient indicates on the recording when symptoms occur and notes any activity, position change, eating, or drinking at the time of the symptom. The data recorded by this portable apparatus is subsequently transferred to a computer for analysis. A fall in pH indicates reflux of acid into the esophagus. Examiners can then determine if the symptoms occur in concert with a reflux event. Sometimes used with an ambulatory heart monitor, this technique helps distinguish cardiac from esophageal chest pain.

Anorectal Manometry

Anorectal manometry is a technique to record the pressures within the rectum and the anal sphincters. The procedure is used to evaluate patients with constipation, fecal incontinence, or unexplained rectal pain (see chapter 11). Patients must discontinue laxatives, anticholinergic drugs, and narcotics at least twenty-four hours prior to the test. They use a phosphate enema one-to-two hours prior to the test, but should report to the clinic prior to bowel cleansing because the presence of stool in the sigmoid colon and rectum is valuable diagnostic information. The procedure is painless, but uncomfortable.

The anus and surrounding skin are tested for sensation; soiling, hemorrhoids, or scar tissue are noted. The patient is asked to squeeze the anal sphincter muscles while the doctor notes the pressure that is generated as he examines the anus. Puborectalis muscle contraction is similarly estimated, and any pain is noted. When the patient strains to defecate, the examiner observes whether the pelvic floor descends and anal canal pressure decreases.

Next, with the patient sitting in a commode chair, the recording apparatus is carefully placed in the anus and lower rectum. This consists of a six-lumen catheter with lateral sensing orifices that open at equal intervals around the circumference. The catheter orifices are perfused with water throughout the procedure. A polyvinyl catheter with a latex balloon on the tip can be filled with air through a central lumen. Four lateral-sensing orifices are assembled at 1-cm intervals below the balloon. Finally the apparatus includes another sensing device that rests in the anal canal to record pelvic floor electromyographic activity. Data from these several sensors are recorded electronically.

Pressures are recorded as the apparatus is withdrawn (*pull-throughs*). Anal pressures are recorded while the patient squeezes the balloon as hard as possible. The balloon is inflated in stages and the patient reports any urge to defecate, as well as any pain. The resulting measurements provide information about anorectal sensation and anus and pelvic-floor muscle power. The demonstration of a failure of the internal anal sphincter to relax in response to balloon distension in the rectum is an important indicator of Hirschprung's disease. The anorectal manometry apparatus may be used in biofeedback training for incontinence or pelvic floor dyssynergia.

Source
Drossman DA, Shaheen NJ, Grimm IS. *Handbook of Gastroenterologic Procedures*, 4th ed. Philadelphia: Lippencott Williams and Wilkins, 2005.

Glossary

abdominal distension: objective evidence that the abdomen is swollen, bloated, or full. Distension may be visible to the patient or to an observer.
abuse: threats or actions of an emotional, sexual, or physical nature in which a power differential exists between the perpetrator and the victim
acetylcholine: an important neurotransmitter that propagates nerve impulses
achalasia: the most readily recognized motor disorder of the esophagus, characterized by aperistalsis of the esophageal body and a failure of the lower esophageal sphincter to relax
adherence: a subject's compliance with a research protocol
adverse event: in this book, an undesirable result of a treatment
aerophagia: ingestion of air. See *Mueller maneuver*.
afferent nerve (afferents): nerve fibers (usually sensory) that carry impulses from an organ or tissue toward the central nervous system; the information processing centers of the enteric nervous system.
aganglionosis: congenital absence of ganglionic cells in the enteric nervous system in a segment of bowel. This may affect the anal canal and is the pathophysiological basis for Hirschprung's disease.
alarm symptoms: symptoms such as fever, bleeding, anemia, and weight loss, or physical findings such as an abdominal mass that cannot be explained by a functional gastrointestinal disorder
allodynia: a form of visceral hypersensitivity in which there is an abnormal pain response to an innocuous or nonnoxious visceral afferent signal
anal endosonography: examination of the anus by placing an ultrasonic transducer/probe into the anal canal and projecting images of the internal and external anal sphincters
anal fissure: tear in the skin or mucosa in or adjacent to the anal canal, causing stinging, severe pain, or itching during defecation
anemia: reduced blood hemoglobin or red cell concentration
anorectal angle: the (approximately) 90-degree angle between the rectum and the anal canal. This angle becomes more obtuse during defecation and more acute when holding back stool. The angle is formed by the contraction of the puborectalis muscle.
anoscopy: examination of the anus and lower rectum with a rigid cone or tube
antidepressant: a class of drugs whose primary effect is to correct neuro-

transmitter imbalance in the central nervous system for the purpose of correcting the symptoms of major depression

antipsychotic: agents that act mainly via dopaminergic pathways in the central nervous system to decrease symptoms of psychosis, such as delusions (including somatic delusions), hallucinations, and severe agitation

antral dysrhythmia: abnormal electrical rhythm in the gastric antrum (bradygastria/tachygastria), analogous to cardiac arrhythmia

anus: opening at the lower extremity of the rectum that is surrounded by muscles known as the internal and external anal sphincters

anxiety: a subjective sense of feeling worried, often accompanied by bodily symptoms, for example, palpitations, breathlessness, abdominal churning; occasionally amounts to panic.

anxiety disorder: excessive anxiety and worry that cannot be controlled and is persistent with a range of symptoms. Mild forms include phobias; more severe forms amount to panic disorder.

anxiolytic: a drug that can decrease, via action on the central nervous system, the symptoms of acute or chronic anxiety, including panic disorder, obsessive-compulsive disorder, phobia, or generalized anxiety

aperistalsis: failure of peristalsis

autonomic nervous system (ANS): regulates individual organ function and homeostasis. For the most part it is not subject to voluntary control.

axons: fibers that carry impulses away from the perikaryon of a nerve cell

bacterial enteritis: bacterial infection of the intestines

behavior: acts, activities, responses to reactions, movements, processes, operations, etc.; in short, any measurable response of an organism.

belch: retrograde expulsion of gas or air (usually ingested) from the upper gut

benzodiazepine: a class of drugs that act on the cerebral cortex and ascending reticular activating system to facilitate the effect of the inhibitor peptide gamma amino butyric acid (GABA), which in turn decreases central nervous system irritability and promotes smooth-muscle relaxation and sleep, and lessens arousal (decreases anxiety)

bile salts and bile acids: cholesterol products of the liver that are secreted in the bile. In the intestines they assist in emulsifying fat, facilitating its absorption. They are reabsorbed from the ileum and recycled through the liver.

bile-salt diarrhea: a condition in which bile salts secreted by the liver are not reabsorbed in the ileum and recycled, but instead enter the colon where they have a laxative effect. The condition occurs if the ileum is removed, diseased, or fails to function normally.

biliary sphincter of Oddi dysfunction: motility abnormalities of the sphincter of Oddi. These include sphincter of Oddi stenosis and sphincter of Oddi dyskinesia.

biliary-type pain (I, II, III): classification of patients with continued biliary-type pain despite cholecystectomy. The classiification is based upon clinical presentation, laboratory results, and endoscopic retrograde cholangiopancreatography (ERCP) findings (chapter 12).

bilirubin: a group of pigments produced by the liver from the hemoglobin that is released from red blood cells at the end of their life span. Pigments excreted in the bile account for the color of stool.

biofeedback: the use of electronic or mechanical devices to provide visual and/or auditory information (feedback) on a biological process for the purpose of teaching an individual to control the biological process

biomedical model: a model of illness and disease in Western medical education and research. Two such models are 1) reductionism- the belief that all conditions can be linearly reduced to a single etiology and 2) dualism- in which illness and disease are dichotomized either to an "organic" disorder having an objectively defined etiology, or a "functional" disorder, with no specific etiology or pathophysiology.

biopsy: surgical procurement of a sample of tissue that, when processed, can be examined by a microscope

biopsychosocial model: a model that proposes that illness and disease result from simultaneously interacting systems at the cellular, tissue, interpersonal, and environmental level. It incorporates the biologic aspects of the disorder with the unique psychosocial features of the individual, and helps explain the variability in symptom expression among individuals having the same biological condition.

bipolar depression: an affective disorder in which the patient may experience both depressive and manic episodes

blinding: a process in which participants in a clinical trial are not aware which treatment they are receiving. When only the subjects are blinded in a randomized controlled trial, it is said to be single-blind. When both subjects and investigators are blinded, the trial is said to be double-blind. Sometimes called "masking."

bloating: the sensation of abdominal distension, with or without objective evidence

borborygmi: audible bowel sounds

brain-gut axis: the bidirectional nervous connections between the brain (central nervous system or CNS) and gut (enteric and autonomic nervous systems) that serve various physiological functions. Visceral afferent fibers project to somatotypic, emotional, and cognitive centers of the CNS, producing a variety of interpretations of stimuli based on prior learning and one's cognitive and emotional state. In turn, the CNS can inhibit or facilitate afferent nociceptive (pain-sensing) signals, motility, secretory function, or inflammation.

Bristol Stool Form Scale: a seven-point descriptor scale of stool form ranging from watery to hard and lumpy. The scale correlates with whole-gut transit time. (See figure 1, chapter 6.)

bulimia: a compulsive eating disorder characterized by ingestion of large amounts of food followed by self-induced vomiting and purgation

bulking agents: macromolecular substances that increase stool bulk and soften feces by water binding. They may be of plant origin (e.g., bran, plantago) or synthetic (e.g., polyethylene glycol). They cannot be split by the enzymes of the human gut, but some may be partially digested by the colon flora.

burp: retrograde expulsion of gas or air (usually ingested) from the upper gut

Carnett's test: a means of determining likely sources of abdominal pain. If the pain increases with abdominal muscle flexion, a muscle wall etiology is indicated (e.g., cutaneous nerve entrapment, a hernia, or a spinal nerve. If the pain is reduced with abdominal muscle flexion the cause is usually visceral.

catastrophizing: thinking that tends to dwell on the worst possible outcome of any situation in which there is a possibility of an unpleasant outcome. (e.g., A person taking an airplane dwells on the possibility of the airplane crashing.)

CCK: cholecystokinin

cecum: the first part of the colon, just beyond the ileocecal valve

celiac (coeliac) disease: a disease of the small intestine characterized by a damaged mucosa; it results in nutritional deficiencies, weight loss, and diarrhea. Healing occurs when gluten is withdrawn from the diet.

cerebral cortex: the grey outer matter of the cerebral hemispheres, consisting of layered masses of nerve cells that perform the higher neurological functions

cholecystectomy: surgical removal of the gallbladder

cholecystokinin: a messenger peptide in the digestive tract that may be released as a hormone from enteroendocrine cells or as a neurotransmitter from enteric neurons

choledochoscintigraphy: quantitative scintigraphic measurement of the time for bile transit from the liver to the duodenum in patients who have undergone cholecystectomy

cholescintigraphy: quantitative scintigraphic measurement of gallbladder emptying after intravenous infusion of CCK

cholestyramine: a powdered resin capable of binding bile salts; it is used to treat bile-salt diarrhea

cholinergic: a class of drugs that produce the same effects as acetylcholine, the most common neurohormone of the parasympathetic nervous system, which is responsible for the everyday work of the body (salivation, digestion, muscle relaxation)

cognitions: beliefs, attitudes, expectations, and other mental events

cognitive behavioral therapy: several approaches or sets of techniques drawn from a large pool of cognitive and behavioral strategies. The theme that unifies these approaches in functional GI disorders centers on an exploration of how certain cognitions and behaviors affect gut symptoms and associated psychosocial distress.

colic: periodic spasmodic pain from hollow organs such as the ureters, bile ducts, and intestines. Contrary to popular belief, biliary pain does not wax and wane. Hence, "biliary colic" is a misnomer.

colonoscopy: examination of the colon through an endoscope

compliance: the capability of a region of the gut to adapt to an increased intraluminal volume. See alternate meaning under *adherence.*

coping: behaviors or mental activities that manage (i.e., master, tolerate, minimize) environmental and internal stressors that tax or exceed a person's resources. They may be adaptive (e.g., problem-focused) or maladaptive (e.g., emotion-focused, "catastrophizing") in terms of health status. Therefore,

coping is a mediating psychosocial factor in illness that may positively or negatively affect health outcome.

corticotropin-releasing factor (CRF): chemical substance released from neurons in the hypothalamus and possibly by enteric neurons; a mediator of physical or emotional stress effects on gastrointestinal tract behavior.

Crohn's disease: inflammatory bowel disease that principally affects the small bowel and colon

cyclic vomiting: recurrent stereotypic episodes of intense nausea and vomiting that last hours to days, separated by symptom-free intervals.

defecography: radiographic assessment of the shape of the rectum during attempted defecation. A mixture of barium sulfate and a thickening agent is inserted into the rectum prior to attempted defecation.

depression: a feeling of pessimism, sadness, tearfulness, and/or irritability

depressive disorders: depression accompanied by reduced activities, suppressed appetite, interrupted sleep patterns, fatigue or loss of energy, and feelings of guilt or worthlessness. Suicidal ideas occur in severe forms.

descending perineum syndrome: greater than normal descent of the perineum during straining at defecation

diabetic peripheral neuropathy: peripheral nerve injury resulting from diabetes

dietary fiber: naturally occurring bulking agents, mostly of plant origin

discomfort: a subjective, unpleasant sensation or feeling that is not interpreted as pain

dissacharidases: enzymes located in the inner surface of the small intestine that split dissacharide sugars such as sucrose and lactose into constituent monsaccharides such as fructose, glucose, and galactose

dissociation: disruption of the usual integration of consciousness, memory, and perception of the environment. This may lead to a number of symptoms including loss of memory, apparent loss of identity, and numerous unexplained bizarre bodily symptoms.

distension: see *abdominal distension*

diverticula, diverticulum: outpouching of the intestine, usually due to a weakness in the wall. In the colon, diverticula appear in older people through the openings where blood vessels pierce the muscle layers. Normally these cause no symptoms. In the small bowel, diverticula can occur spontaneously, usually in the duodenum.

diverticulitis: damage caused by the bursting of a colon diverticulum

dorsal root ganglion: the location of cell bodies of spinal afferent neurons

dualism: a concept first proposed by Descartes that separates mind and body. Cartesian dualism (the biomedical model) is the dominant model of disease in Western culture, and is challenged by the biopsychosocial model.

duodenum: the first or proximal portion of the small intestine

dyschezia: difficult defecation, defined by straining, a feeling of incomplete evacuation, and/or digital facilitation of defecation (pressing around the anus or inside the vagina)

dysmotility: disturbed intestinal motility

dyspepsia: pain or discomfort centered in the upper abdomen
dysphagia: a sensation of abnormal bolus transit through the esophageal body
dyssynergic defecation (also pelvic floor dyssynergia, anismus, spastic pelvic floor syndrome): a chronic disorder of defecation that is due to functional outlet obstruction by paradoxical puborectalis muscle and/or contraction of the external anal sphincter

early satiety: a feeling that the stomach is overfilled soon after starting to eat. The sensation is out of proportion to the size of the meal being eaten, so that the meal cannot be finished.
ECRP: see *endoscopic retrograde cholangiopancreatography*
efferent nerves (efferents): nerve fibers that carry impulses away from the central nervous system, causing muscles to contract and glands to secrete (inhibitory efferent nerves)
electrical slow waves: omnipresent form of electrical activity (rhythmic depolarization and repolarization) in gastrointestinal muscle cells
electrogalvanic stimulation: transrectal low-frequency electrical stimulation that is used to treat rectal pain by relaxing skeletal muscles in the pelvic floor
electrogastrography: the recording of gastric electrical activity from surface electrodes positioned on the abdominal wall
electromyography (EMG): recording of the electrical potentials that are generated by muscle cells when they contract
emotion-focused coping: a method in which an individual seeks to manage the distressing emotions evoked by a situation or condition (e.g., praying or denial)
encopresis: perverse, voluntary withholding of stool, usually by children, mentally handicapped, or senile people. See *stool withholding*.
endoscopic retrograde cholangiopancreatography (ECRP): a procedure that is used to visualize the biliary tree. An endoscope is passed through the stomach and its side-viewing tip is positioned opposite the sphincter of Oddi. A special cannula is passed through the endoscope and into the bile or pancreatic duct. Radiopaque liquid is then injected into the ducts so they can be viewed on an x-ray screen
endoscopy: examination of the inside of the gastrointestinal tract using an instrument that is passed through the mouth or anus. The image is transmitted to the eye by fiber optics, or via a chip to a TV monitor. Biopsies and other procedures may be conducted through the instrument. Endoscopy includes esophagoscopy, gastroscopy, esophagogastroduodenoscopy, and enteroscopy via the mouth, and anoscopy, sigmoidoscopy, and colonoscopy via the anus.
endosonography: use of a device passed through an endoscope that transmits sound waves to demonstrate body tissues
enkephalins: a family of natural chemical painkillers that act on receptor sites for alkaloids from the opium poppy in the human brain, affording pain relief as a body defense
enteric minibrain: a reference to the brain-like functions of the enteric nervous system
enteric nervous system: the part of the autonomic nervous system that is situated

within the walls of the digestive tract and is involved with independent integrative neural control of digestive functions

enterocele: the descent of loops of the small intestine into the pelvis that bulge into the vagina during straining. An enterocele may cause pain and/or obstructed defecation.

enteroscopy: examination of the small intestine through a specially designed endoscope

epigastric: pertaining to the area of the upper abdomen immediately below the breastbone and between the lowest ribs

epithelial barrier: a wall formed by "tight junctions" between epithelial cells of the gastrointestinal mucosa. The barrier prevents the translocation of infectious agents and large molecules from the gut lumen into the body.

erythrocyte sedimentation rate (ESR): the rate at which blood cells settle in a vertical tube. A rapid ESR is a nonspecific sign of inflammation and other diseases.

esophagitis: inflammation of the esophagus, most commonly due to gastric acid reflux

esophagogastroduodenoscopy: examination of the esophagus, stomach, and proximal duodenum through an endoscope

esophagoscopy: examination of the esophagus through an endoscope

etiology: cause or origin of a disease or disorder

external anal sphincter: a ring of skeletal muscle surrounding the anal canal that can be voluntarily contracted to postpone defecation

fecal impaction: larger than normal, firm mass of stool in the rectum or colon that is difficult for the person to evacuate. This may contribute to fecal incontinence (overflow).

fecaloma: a mass of hard stool in the rectum; fecal impaction

fart: to pass gas per the anus; the act, sound, or odor of gas passing per the rectum.

fever: body temperature in excess of 37 degrees Celsius (98.6 degrees Fahrenheit)

flatulence: usually a euphemism for farting, but may embrace gassiness, bloating, even belching. Therefore, it is a term of little value.

flatus: gas (wind) passed per the anus

fructose: a natural sugar; a monosaccharide that, combined with glucose, constitutes sucrose, or table sugar. It occurs naturally in fruits, honey, and chocolate. When ingested in excess it can cause diarrhea.

fullness: an unpleasant sensation like the persistence of food in the stomach that may or may not occur postprandially

functional: pertaining to a presumed disorder of function, used in this book to describe gastrointestinal syndromes for which no pathology or pathophysiology is recognized. (Opposite of "organic.")

functional magnetic resonance imaging (fMRI): the use of MRI to measure the blood flow changes that occur during neural activity in the brain or spinal cord.

functional outlet obstruction: inability or difficulty to void the rectum due to pelvic floor dyssynergia, internal prolapse, or enterocele that becomes apparent only upon straining

functional somatic syndromes: functional syndromes attributable to a body system

ganglia: a grouping of nerve cell bodies situated outside the central nervous system
ganglionated plexus: an array of ganglia and interganglionic fiber tracts forming parts of the enteric nervous system
gas: known as *wind* in the U.K. In this book, gas refers to the gases in or escaping from the gut.
gastritis: inflammation of the lining of the stomach
gastrocolonic response: activation of intestinal motility in response to a meal
gastroduodenum: stomach and duodenum
gastroesophageal reflux (GER): the retrograde flow of gastric contents into the esophagus
gastrointestinal motility: the organized application of forces of muscle contraction that results in physiologically significant movement of intraluminal contents
gastroparesis: paralysis (lack of motor activity) of the stomach
gastroscopy: examination of the stomach using an endoscope
genetic polymorphism: multiple forms of the same gene
giardiasis: chronic parasitic infection of the small bowel causing diarrhea and weight loss
globus (globus pharyngis, globus pharyngeus): a sensation of something stuck or of a lump or tightness in the throat
gluten: a wheat protein responsible for celiac disease in susceptible people
gut: the gastrointestinal tract, including the esophagus and stomach
gut brain: the enteric nervous system
gut hypersensitivity: an ambiguous term referring to both conscious perception of gut stimuli and to afferent input within gastrointestinal sensory pathways, whether related to perception or to reflex responses. See *visceral hypersensitivity*.

health beliefs (health concerns): patients' beliefs about the causes of illness and worries that they may have a disease
health-related quality of life (HRQOL): the impact that illness has on quality of life, including the individual's perception of his/her illness
heartburn: episodic retrosternal burning; also called pyrosis.
***Helicobacter pylori*:** bacteria residing within the wall of the stomach that cause chronic gastritis and predispose the individual to gastric and duodenal ulcers
hemoglobin: the oxygen-carrying protein in red cells
holism: from the Greek holos, or whole, an approach proposed by Plato, Aristotle, and Hippocrates in ancient Greece. It postulates that mind and body are inseparable, so the study of medical disease must take into account the whole person rather than merely the diseased part. This concept fell into disfavor after Descartes proposed the separation between mind ("res cogitans") and body ("res extensa"). (See *dualism*.)

5-hydroxytryptamine (serotonin), 5-HT: an important neurotransmitter in both central (brain and spinal cord) and peripheral (enteric nervous system) digestive neurophysiology

hyperalgesia: a form of visceral hypersensitivity where there is an increased pain response to a noxious stimulus

hyperpolarization: an increase in negative electrical potential across cell membranes

hypervigilance: intensified attention to/or focus on specific things

hypnosis: a state of focused attention and heightened suggestibility that can be induced in a variety of ways

hypnotherapy: the use of hypnosis to improve psychological and/or physical symptoms. Hypnosis renders patients more responsive to suggestions for symptom improvement.

hypochondriasis: fear of disease (disease phobia), combined with the conviction that one has a disease, in the absence of objective evidence that disease is present

ileocecal valve: muscular thickening at the distal (far) end of the ileum where it empties intestinal contents into the colon

ileum: the last of the three segments of the small intestine

illness behavior: conduct or behavior in response to an individual's perceptions of being ill or not well. Examples include visits to the doctor, taking time off work, staying in bed, and taking medications. This behavior is not necessarily an abnormal reaction to illness but a behavioral response based on a person's formulation and attribution of his/her illness.

incidence: occurrence of an illness or disease, often expressed as the number of cases occurring in a defined population within a year

incident cases: those who have sought health care for a condition for the first time in the past year. (Incidence and prevalence are only meaningful when referring to population-based studies.)

indigestion: term used by patients for an unpleasant abdominal or substernal sensation from such a variety of illnesses that it is of no use diagnostically. Further symptom description is needed.

inflammatory bowel disease: chronic inflammatory conditions of unknown cause affecting the intestines. They include ulcerative colitis and Crohn's disease.

innervated: describes a structure that is supplied with intact nerves

interganglionic fiber tracts: bundles of nerve fibers connecting adjacent ganglia of the enteric nervous system

interpersonal therapy: a form of psychotherapy in which the therapist identifies aspects of the relationship between the patient and the therapist that mirror difficulties in relationships outside of the therapy

intussusception: telescoping of any part of the intestine or rectum

jejunum: the middle segment of the small intestine

lactose intolerance: diarrhea and excessive intestinal gas due to a failure of digestion of lactose in the small intestine, which in turn is due to an insufficiency of the enzyme lactase in the small intestine

laxative: a compound that increases fecal water content. The primary mechanism is the inhibition of colonic water absorption or stimulation of active or passive colonic water secretion. Some laxatives are also prokinetics, and prokinetics can be laxative.

laxative abuse: laxative ingestion without proper indication or at higher than necessary doses

learned illness behavior: patterning of pain behavior during childhood by parental modeling

life stress: stressful events that are part of life but occur rarely, e.g., bereavement, divorce, severe financial loss, severe illness in a family member, serious accident, etc.

macrolide antibiotics: a group of antibiotics exemplified by erythromycin and clarithromycin

Manning criteria: early symptom criteria for the irritable bowel syndrome developed in the late 1970s

manometric: pertaining to pressure measurements (in this context, within the gut lumen)

manometry: use of pressure sensors within a hollow organ such as the esophagus to measure changes that reflect the organ's muscle contractions

marker test: test of whole-gut transit time. Ingested small radiopaque markers are followed through the gastrointestinal tract.

mask: see *blinding*

mechanical obstruction: any physical obstacle to the forward movement of intestinal contents, including tumors, scar tissue, or volvulus (twisting). Mechanical obstruction is distinguished from a functional obstruction, which is due to absent or abnormal contractions of the intestine.

megarectum: abnormal enlargement of the rectum

metiorism: *archaic.* flatulent dyspepsia with gas in the alimentary canal

morning rush syndrome: urgent diarrhea upon arising

motility: movements within the intestinal tract, encompassing the phenomena of contractile activity, myoelectrical activity, tone, compliance, wall tension, and transit within the gastrointestinal tract

motor neuron: a nerve cell that sends an axon to a muscle or, by extension, any effector cell or organ

mucosa: cellular lining of the intestines or other hollow organs

mucosal plexus: a gathering of nerve cell bodies lying beneath the mucosa; part of the enteric nervous system.

Mueller maneuver: deep inspiration against a closed glottis

myenteric plexus: ganglionated plexus of the enteric nervous system situated between the longitudinal and circular muscle coats of the muscularis externa of the digestive tract; also called Auerbach's plexus.

myogenic: originating in muscle tissue

myopathic pseudoobstruction: pathologic failure of propulsion in the gastrointestinal tract related to muscular degeneration and weakened contractility

nausea: queasiness or sick sensation; a feeling of the need to vomit.
neural networks: aggregates of interconnected neurons that produce a range of behaviors associated with the central and enteric nervous systems
neurogastroenterology: a subdiscipline of gastroenterology that encompasses all basic and clinical aspects of nervous system involvement in normal and disordered digestive functions and sensations
neurogenic inflammation: inflammation initiated by activity in sensory nerves and the release of substance P
neurokinin A: a neurotransmitter
neuropathic pseudoobstruction: pathologic failure of propulsion in the gastrointestinal tract related to enteric neuropathy and loss of nervous control mechanisms
neuroticism: a personality trait characterized by a predisposition to experience anxiety, depression, anger, and a sense of hopelessness and helplessness about the future (negative affect)
neurotransmitter: substance released from nerve cells at synapses that amounts to a chemical signal from one neuron to another or from motor neurons to effectors
nitric oxide: a putative inhibitory neurotransmitter that is released by enteric motor neurons to gastrointestinal muscles
nitroglycerine: a pharmaceutical that is placed under the tongue to relieve angina pectoris (reversible heart pain due to insufficient blood supply to the heart muscle)
nociception: the experience of a stimulus as harmful, in contrast to a pleasant sensation
nonpatients: in this book, those who have never sought health care for their functional gastrointestinal disorders

obsessive-compulsive disorder: an anxiety disorder characterized by recurrent, intrusive thoughts and compulsive, stereotyped, repetitive behaviors or cognitions
obstipation: severe constipation
'on-demand' treatment: period of treatment in which the patient initiates therapy during a time when symptoms are present
operant conditioning: a behavior therapy in which a response is reinforced or suppressed by immediate reward or punishment
organic: in this book, pertaining to diseases or disorders for which an anatomic or physiological cause is known. (Opposite of "functional.")
over-the-counter: pertains to a medication available in pharmacies or grocery stores that does not require a doctor's prescription

pain-prone personality: constellation of personality features, including personality disorders, exhibited by patients whose lives are dominated by pain. Common characteristics include childhood abuse or deprivation, a history of pain-related surgeries, care-seeking from multiple physicians, and disappointment with therapeutic results.

pancreaticobiliary tree: the branching bile and pancreatic ducts leading from the liver and pancreas to the duodenum

paradoxical sphincter contraction: contraction of the external anal sphincter and/or the puborectalis muscle upon straining, which in turn impedes stool passage. Causes are painful anal disorders (fissures, perianal thrombosis, abscess) or pelvic floor dyssynergia.

parasympathetic: pertaining to a division of the autonomic nervous system with its outflow from the central nervous system into certain cranial and sacral nerves and having its ganglia in or near the innervated viscera

patients: in this book, people with symptoms of functional gastrointestinal disease (FGID) who have ever sought health care for them

pelvic floor dyssynergia: failure of coordination of the muscles of the pelvic floor during defecation

pelvic pain: a term used by gynecologists to describe pain in the lower abdomen. It is not clear where the pelvis begins and the abdomen begins. For clarity, and to avoid suggesting etiology, "lower abdominal pain" is preferred.

pelvic tension myalgia: a synonym for levator ani syndrome (See appendix A, F2a.1. for a description of this syndrome, or refer to chapter 11.)

perineum: that part of the pelvic floor that lies between the tops of the thighs and in front of the anus

peristalsis: coordinated intestinal smooth-muscle contractions preceded by relaxation that move intestinal contents along; also occurs in the esophagus, stomach, and hollow tubes in the genitourinary tract such as the ureters.

personality disorder: an enduring pattern of inner experience and behavior that deviates markedly from the expectations of the individual's culture. It is persistent, starts in adolescence, is stable over time, and is not amenable to psychiatric treatment.

phobia: an anxiety disorder characterized by a) persistent fear of a specific situation out of proportion to the reality of the danger; b) compelling desire to avoid and escape the situation; c) recognition that fear is unreasonably excessive; d) it is not due to any other disorder.

physician-patient relationship (physician-patient interaction): ideally understood in terms of interpersonal behaviors that enhance or diminish mutual communication, satisfaction, and trust. In particular, physician behaviors may enhance or diminish this interaction. Positive physician behaviors are characterized by empathy, respect, and positive regard.

placebo: pill, injection, sham incision, or other harmless and ineffective treatment. Used in the past as a treatment to "harmlessly" please the patient, the term is now commonly used to describe a control treatment in a randomized clinical trial.

placebo effect: in randomized clinical trials, the difference in outcome between a placebo-treated group and an untreated group in an unbiased experiment. In clinical practice, change in a patient's illness attributable to the symbolic import of the treatment rather than a specific pharmacologic or physiologic property.

placebo response: response to a treatment that is the sum of the placebo effect, the natural history of the disease being tested, parallel treatments, and time-dependent factors such as regression to the mean

polyp: a protuberance from an epithelial surface; in the colon, commonly comprising neoplastic tissue that is usually benign, but may be precancer or cancer.

positive emission tomography (PET): a nuclear medicine medical imaging technique that produces a three-dimensional image or map of functional processes in the body

postprandial: after meals

prevalence: existing number of cases of a disease or disorder

prevalent cases: in this book, those who have ever sought health care for their FGIDs

probiotics: living microorganisms that, upon ingestion in certain numbers, exert health benefits beyond general nutrition

problem-based coping: a method in which an individual tries to deal directly with situational stressors by changing the stressor or oneself (e.g., by seeking social support, reappraising the stressor, etc.). In general, problem-based coping is used in situations that are appraised by patients to be changeable or adaptable, and is an appropriate coping method for chronic illness.

proctalgia fugax: fleeting pains (only a few minutes in duration) in the rectum or anal canal, in the absence of known organic etiology

progressive muscle relaxation: voluntary relaxation through systematically tensing and relaxing different muscle groups while attending to the sensations associated with tension and relaxation

prokinetic: pertains to drugs that act on enteric nerve endings to enhance propulsion of contents through the gut. Such a drug may act by direct muscle stimulation, release of motor neurotransmitters, or blockade of inhibitory neurotransmitters.

pseudodiarrhea: frequent and/or urgent defecations of normal or firm/lumpy stools

pseudoobstruction: pathologic failure of propulsion in the gastrointestinal tract in the absence of mechanical obstruction

psychiatric diagnosis: a diagnosis of one of the psychiatric disorders (standardized in the *Diagnostic and Statistical Manual IV* (DSM IV) and the *World Health Organization International Classification of Diseases*)

psychodynamic therapy: the application of psychological theories derived from the works of Freud and others. The theories base current problems on past difficulties in relationships, especially with parents.

psychological distress: symptoms of anxiety or depression not amounting to anxiety or depressive disorders

psychological state: a temporary or changeable phenomenon, e.g., anxiety

psychological traits: personality characteristics or an internal predisposition to respond in a particular way

psychoneuroendocrinology: the study of the interrelationship between environmental stress and neuroendocrine functions

psychopharmacology: the study of drugs to treat symptoms of psychiatric disease

psychophysiology: the study of the interactions between psychological factors (e.g., anxiety, stress) and physiological factors (e.g., muscle tension, cardiovascular arousal)

psychosomatic: pertaining to medical diseases that are believed to be caused by a pre-existent biologic susceptibility and disease-specific psychological characteristics

psychotherapist: an individual who engages in behavioral treatment of emotional distress using various modalities, including hypnosis, relaxation training, and traditional talk therapy

puborectalis muscle: a sling muscle that anchors to the symphysis pubis anteriorily and loops around the rectum to form the anorectal angle. This muscle is important to fecal continence.

pudendal nerve terminal motor latency: the time between electrical stimulation of the pudendal nerve with electrodes on the tip of a gloved finger, and the contraction of the external anal sphincter. It is used as a measure of the integrity of the pudendal nerve.

pylorus: the muscular ring or valve at the junction of the stomach and the duodenum

pyrosis: heartburn

quality of life (QOL): a person's perception that he is able to meet his needs in self-care, physical activities, work and social interactions, and psychological well-being

radiograph: an x-ray-generated image

receptor (membrane): cell membrane surface proteins with a unique structure that permits the binding of specific chemical signal substances, which triggers changes in the cell's behavior

rectal prolapse: protrusion of the mucosal lining of the rectum through the anus

rectocele: weakness in the tissues surrounding the rectum that permits it to bulge abnormally. The most common rectocele is one affecting the rectovaginal septum in women.

rectum: the lowest segment of the colon, located within the pelvis and terminated at the anus

reflex: a neuronal event that occurs beyond volition. In neurophysiology, a relatively simple behavioral response of an effector that is produced by influx of sensory afferent impulses to a neural center, and its reflection as efferent impulses back to the periphery to the effector (e.g., muscle). The neural center may consist of interneurons. The simplest reflex circuit consists only of sensory and motor neurons.

Rome **criteria:** lists of symptoms among which a specified minimum number allows a diagnosis of a functional gastrointestinal disorder

rumination: a regurgitation of recently ingested food into the mouth with subsequent remastication and reswallowing or spitting out. The regurgitation is effortless, unassociated with abdominal discomfort, heartburn, or nausea, and sometimes seems to be a pleasurable experience.

scintigraphic techniques: the use of radioisotopes either ingested with food or released from swallowed capsules. In gastroenterology, such techniques are used to measure transit times through different regions of the gastrointestinal tract.

scybala: hard, round, lumpy stools

secretomotor neuron: motor neurons in the submucous plexus that innervate and evoke secretion from the intestinal glands

self-esteem: a personality trait whereby an individual is able to evaluate his/her abilities, achievements, and value in society in a way that promotes confidence and personal satisfaction

sensory neuron: a neuron that conducts impulses that arise in a sense organ or at sensory nerve endings

sensory receptor: a cell or part of a cell that is specialized to convert environmental stimuli into nerve impulses or a response that in turn evokes nerve impulses. Most sensory receptor cells are nerve cells, but other cells can be receptors (e.g., intestinal enteroendocrine cells). One method of classifying receptors is by their unique stimulus. Chemoreceptors, osmoreceptors, and mechanoreceptors are normally stimulated by chemicals, osmotic pressure differences, and mechanical events, respectively.

sigmoid colon: an s-shaped segment of colon above the rectum

sigmoidoscopy: endoscopic examination of the anus, rectum, and sigmoid colon through an endoscope

somatization: the behavior of reporting physical symptoms that are not associated with any known pathophysiological process, or that are excessive when compared to known pathophysiology

sorbitol: artificial sugar used in "calorie-free" chewing gum and confections. In sufficient quantity, it may cause diarrhea and is used as a laxative.

specific thalamocortical projection: a sensory pathway from the periphery to the cerebral cortex that involves only two synaptic connections

sphincter of Oddi: the muscular valve at the duodenal end of the common bile duct. The valve commonly includes the end of the pancreatic duct as well.

steatorrhea: abnormally high levels of fat in the stool

stethoscope sign: abdominal tenderness on palpation that is not evident when similar pressure is applied during auscultation with a stethoscope, suggesting a functional source

stool withholding: a condition in which a child attempts to delay the act of defecation by contracting the pelvic floor and the gluteal muscle after having experienced a painful or frightening defecation. It is the most common cause of functional constipation in children. (See *encopresis*.)

stress: any external or internal stimulus or sequence of stimuli that tend to disrupt homeostasis. It may be an environmental stress or the feeling of being stressed. Stress results in disease when mechanisms of homeostatic adjustment fail.

substance P: a neurotransmitter

surfactant: a substance that reduces surface tension and promotes wetting of surfaces. Sometimes a surfactant is included in antacids in a doubtful attempt to treat "flatulence."

sympathetic: pertaining to a division of the autonomic nervous system with its outflow from the central nervous system in the thoracolumbar segments of the spinal cord. The celiac, superior, and inferior mesenteric ganglia are parts of the sympathetic nervous system that are found in the abdomen.

synapse: a connection between neurons consisting of a presynaptic site of chemical transmitter release and a postsynaptic site of action of the released transmitter

tachykinin: a neurotransmitter

therapeutic gain: the (usually beneficial) effect on a patient's symptom or pathological abnormality of the treatment itself, which may be a drug, a diet, a device, a procedure or a psychological treatment. It is also called the delta, or the absolute benefit increase.

thyrotropin-releasing hormone: a hormone in the hypothalamic-pituitary axis that also functions as a neurotransmitter at synapses in the dorsal vagal complex in the brain stem

tonic contraction: a degree of tension, firmness, or maintained contraction in a muscle

transit time: the time taken for food or other material to traverse a specified region of the gut

tropical sprue: a disease of the small intestine caused by bacteria that leads to malabsorption among people living for long periods in the tropics

ulcerative colitis: chronic inflammatory bowel disease of the colon

vago-vagal reflex: a reflex for which both afferent and efferent fibers are contained in the vagus nerves

vasoactive intestinal peptide: a possible inhibitory neurotransmitter released by enteric musculomotor neurons to gastrointestinal muscles

villous adenoma: a particular neoplastic polyp in the colon that is often premalignant or even malignant. Large villous tumors of the lower colon produce large volumes of fluid that may be mistaken for diarrhea.

visceral hyperalgesia: see *visceral hypersensitivity*

visceral hypersensitivity: gut hypersensitivity; a condition in which the individual responses to visceral afferent signals are amplified or increased. It is the appreciation of unpleasant gut symptoms elicited by stimuli (such as balloon distension of the gut) that would ordinarily not be noticed or considered noxious.

wall tension: the force acting on the gut wall that results from the interaction between intraluminal content and the reaction of the muscular and elastic properties of the wall

whole-gut transit time: the time required for transit of intestinal contents from mouth to anus

wind: a colloquial term for flatus in the U.K., like *gas* in North America

Resources

Functional Gastrointestinal Support Groups

International Foundation for Functional Gastrointestinal Disorders (IFFGD)
P.O. Box 170864
Milwaukee, WI 53217-8076
Toll-free telephone: 888-964-2001
E-mail: iffgd@iffgd.org
Web site: www.iffgd.org

Canadian Society of Intestinal Research
855 West 12th Avenue
Vancouver, BC V5Z 1M9
Toll-free phone: 866-600-4875
Fax: 604-875-4429
E-mail: info@badgut.com
Web site: http://www.badgut.com/

Cyclic Vomiting Syndrome Association (CVSA)
2819 West Highland Boulevard
Milwaukee, WI 53208
Telephone: 414-342-7880
Fax: 414-342-8980
E-mail: cvsa@cvsaonline.org

UNC Center for Functional GI & Motility Disorders
CB #7080, Bioinformatics Building
University of North Carolina
Chapel Hill, NC 27599-7080
Fax: 919 966-8929
Email: knyrop@med.unc.edu

IBS Network
Unit 5
53 Mowbray Street
Sheffield S3 8EN
United Kingdom
Telephone: 0114 272 32 53
E-mail: info@ibsnetwork.org.uk

ANEMGI-Onlus.
Associazione per la Neurogastroenterologia e la Motilità Gastrointestinale
E-mail: anemgi@anemgi.org
Web site: www.anemgi.org

Books

Drossman DA, Corazziari E, Delvaux M, Spiller RC, Talley NJ, Thompson WG, Whitehead WE, eds., *Rome III: The Functional Gastrointestinal Disorders.* McLean, VA: Degnon Associates Inc.; 2006.

Drossman DA, Shaheen NJ, Grimm IS. *Handbook of Gastroenterologic Procedures,* 4th ed. Philadelphia: Lippincott Williams and Wilkins; 2005.

Lackner JM. *Controlling IBS the Drug-Free Way: A 10-Step Plan for Symptom Relief.* New York: Stewart, Tabori & Chang; 2007.

Talley NJ. *Conquering Irritable Bowel Syndrome.* Hamilton, ON: B. C. Decker, Inc.; 2005.

Thompson WG. *The Placebo Effect: Combining Science and Compassionate Care.* Amherst, NY: Prometheus Books; 2005.

Thompson WG, Heaton KW. *Fast Facts: Irritable Bowel Syndrome,* 2nd ed. Oxford: Health Press; 2003.

Index

Page numbers in italics refer to figures and tables.

abortion, risk of with misoprostil (Cytotec), 155, 171
abuse (sexual or physical), 34, *47,* 108
acetylcholine, 26, 31, 33
achalasia, 32, 169, 205
acid instillation, 84
allodynia, 29, 37
amino acids, 24
ANEMGI-Onlus, 226
angina pectoris, 78
angiograms, 83–84
anorectum, 23, 25, *26,* 33
    anorectum expelling barium (defecography), 90, 93
antidepressants, 146, 152, 169–70
    selective serotonin reuptake inhibitors (SSRIs), 146, 168
        fluoxetine, 151
        paroxitine, 152, 169
        sertraline, 146
    serotonin neurepinephrine reuptake inhibitors (SNRIs), 169
    trazadone, 146
    tricyclic antidepressants, 64, 102, 146
        amitriptyline (Elavil), 151, 169
        desipramine (Norpramin), 152, 169
        doxepin, 151
        nortriptyline (Pamelor), 151, 169
antitissue transglutaminase (tTG-IgA), 70

anus, 26, 90
    anorectal manometry, 205–06
    external anal sphincter, 25, 30
        weakness of, 90
    internal anal sphincter, 25, 30
    ultrasound of, 90
    See also functional anorectal disorders
anxiety, 72, 99, 103, 108, 113
autonomic nervous system, 26
    divisions of, 26–27
        enteric, 26, *27*
        parasympathetic, 26, *27*
        sympathetic, 26, *27*
axons, 27

bacteria, 36–37, 170–71
    anaerobic, 24
    as a cause of chronic diarrhea, 71
    number of intestinal bacteria, 24
bacterial enteritis, 37
belching disorders, 94–95, 98
    aerophagia, 94–95
        Rome III diagnostic criteria for adults, 186
    excessive belching, 95
        Rome III diagnostic criteria for adults, 186
    "supragastric belching," 94
    See also belching disorders, treatment of
belching disorders, treatment of, 150
    chlordiazepoxide drugs, 150
        diazepam (Valium), 150
    sedatives/relaxants, 150
bile, 24

bile salts, 24, 70, 71
  absorption of, 156
  bile salt diarrhea, 70
bilirubin, 24
biofeedback, 143, 159, 160–61, 172–73
"biomarker," 12
Blackman, Carlar, xvi
bloating. *See* functional bloating
borborygmi, 98
brain, 28–29, *29*
  and the cerebral cortex, 103
Bristol Stool Form Scale, 51, *51*, 60, 61, 67, 69, 159
Brody, H., 112

calcium carbonate, 83
Campylobacter, 37
Canadian Society of Intestinal Research, 225
carbon dioxide, 24, 98
celiac disease, 35–36, 54–55, 70, 72
central nervous system (CNS), 28
Chang, Lin, xvii
cholera bacteria, 23
clinical trials. *See* randomized clinical trials (RCTs)
Clostridium botulinin, 168
Clostridium difficile, 164, 170
cognitive behavioral therapy, 143, 172
  and chest pain, 146–47
  and FAPS, 102, 157
  and irritable bowel syndrome (IBS), 153
colon, 22, 23–24, *23*, 30, 35, 201–02
  bacteria in, 36–37
  cancer of, 53, 54, 65, 67, 201
  sigmoid colon, 90
  and water absorption/exchange, 23–24
computed tomography (CT), 53, 98, 204
constipation, 23, 32, 33, 41, 51, *63*, 98, 154, 201. *See also* functional constipation
Crohn's disease, 43–44, 50, 54, 64, 71, 89, 201

Cyclic Vomiting Syndrome Association, 225

defecography, *63*, 90, 93, 204
Degnon, George, xvi
dementia, 89
depression, 34, 35, *47*, 48, 108, 113
  and functional abdominal pain syndrome (FAPS), 103
  and functional bloating, 99
  and functional constipation, 62
  and irritable bowel syndrome (IBS), 55, 56
Descartes, René, 7
diabetes, 6, 17, 89
  diabetic neuropathy, 156
"diagnosis of exclusion," 9
diarrhea, 23, 32, 33, 34, 36, 41, 51, 57, 90
  pseudodiarrhea, 51, 69
  as a risk factor for fecal incontinence, 159
  See also functional diarrhea
disaccharidases, 22
disaccharides, 22
disease
  determining prevalence of, 12–13
  diagnosis of during the Enlightenment, 4
  incidence ("attack rate") of, 12
  prevalence of, 12
  See also disease/illness distinction
disease/illness distinction, 5–6, 122–23
  and the biopsychosocial model, 6–8
  multifactorial nature of, 7
  and reductionism, 7
diverticula, 54
diverticulitis, 54, 64
Dotevall, Gerhard, xv
Drossman, Douglas, xv, xvii, 7, 13, 153
drugs, 113, 128, 131
  analgesics, 124, 157
  aspirin, 148, 157
  antacids, 83, 147, 163–64

Index   229

aluminum/magnesium
    hydroxide combination, 163
calcium carbonate (TUMS), 163
with alginate (Gaviscon), 164
with simethicone, 163
antibiotics, 98–99
    amoxicillin, 165
    clarithromycin, 165
    erythromycin, 149, 166
    metronidazole, 165
anticholinergics, 166–67
    atropine, 156, 159, 167
    cimetropium, 167
    dicyclomine, 146, 167
    hyocyamine, 167
    octilium, 167
antiemetics, 150
antinausea drugs, 150
    diphenhydramine, 150
    ondansetron, 150
antiulcer drugs, 164–65
    bismuth citrate (DeNol), 149, 164
    misoprostol (Cytotec), 164
    sucralfate (Sulcrate), 164
beta adrenergic antagonists, 160
    salbutamol, 160
calcium channel-blocking drugs, 64
    nifedipine, 146
    pinavarium, 167
chloride channel activators, 152
    lubiprostone, 152
diazepam (Valium), 150, 157
histamine H$_2$ antagonists, 164
    cimetidine, 164
    famotidine, 164
    nizatidine, 164
    ranitidine, 164
irritable bowel syndrome, approved drugs for treatment of, *144*
laxatives, 168, 171
    anthraquinone derivatives, 171
    bisacodyl, 155, 171
    calcium polycarbophil, 171
    glycerin suppositories, 171
    lubiprostone (Amitiza), 155, 171

milk of magnesia, 155
misoprosto l (Cytotec), 155
phenolphthalein, 171
polyethylene glycol (PEG
    [CoLyte; GoLYTELy; Peglyte]), 155, 171, 202
saline laxatives, 171
sodium picosulfate, 171
tegaserod (Zelnorm), 152
nonsteroidal anti-inflammatory
    drugs (NSAIDs), 64, 78, 81, 148, 157, 164
opiate antagonists
    trimebutiine, 167
opiates/opioids, 64, 156
    codeine, 156
    diphenoxylate (Lomotil), 156, 159
    loperamide, 156
    tincture of opium, 156
probiotics, 98–99, 170–71
    Bifidobacter, 170
    Lactobacilli, 170
prokinetics, 148–49, 165–66
    cisapride (Propulsid), 148–49, 166
    domperidone (Motilium), 166, 148
    erythromycin, 149, 166
    metoclopramide (Reglan; Maxeran), 148, 165
    side effects of, 165
    tegaserod (Zelnorm), 143, 149, 152, 154, 155, 166, 168
prostaglandin-inhibiting aspirin, 78
proton pump inhibitors (benzimidazoles), 164, 165
    adverse effects of, 164
    esomeprazole (Nexium), 164
    lansoprazole (Prevacid), 164
    omeprazole (Losec; Prilosic), 164
    pantoprazole (Pantozol), 164
    rabeprazole (Pariet), 164
serotonin analogues, 168
    alosetron (Lotronex), 143, 152, 159, 168

drugs (continued)
  serotonin agonists
    sumatriptan (Imitrex), 151
  smooth muscle relaxants (antispasmodics), 151–52, 166–67
    botulinum toxin, 146, 158, 160, 168–69
    mebeverine, 167
  See also antidepressants; placebo effect
dualism, 7
duodenal ulcer, 165, 200–01
dysmotility, 5, 79
dyspepsia, 22, 37, 41, 98, 163
  dysmotility-like, 75, 77
  prevalence of, 14
  reflux-like, 75
  subtypes of, 149
  ulcer-like, 75, 77
  See also functional dyspepsia (non-ulcer dyspepsia)

Engel, George, 7
endoscopic retrograde cholangiopancreatography (ERCP), 104, 105, 158, 201
endoscopy. See functional gastrointestinal diseases, tests for the investigation of
enemas, 155
  barium, 204
  phosphate (Fleet), 155, 202
  small-bowel, 203–04
enteric nervous system (ENS), 26–28, 27, 28, 31, 56–57
  and the brain-gut axis, 28–29, 29
  as the "gut brain," 26, 27
  neurotransmitters found in, 28, 28, 33
epidemiology, 12, 77
epigastric pain syndrome (EPS), 75, 81, 147
  response of to medication, 149
  Rome III diagnostic criteria for adults, 186
epiphenomena, 5
esophagitis, 83, 85

esophagus, 20–21, 21, 30, 33, 37, 169, 204
  disorders of, 41–42
  lower esophageal sphincter (LES), 20–21, 21, 28, 30, 31, 32, 94
    paradoxical relaxation of, 96–97
  motility of, 205
  upper esophageal sphincter, 20, 30, 33
  See also functional esophageal disorders
European Agency for the Evaluation of Medicinal Products (EMEA), 128

fatty acids, 24
  short-chain, 24
fibromyalgia, 56, 103
functional abdominal pain syndrome (FAPS), 99–103
  affective-motivational component of, 102, 124
  characteristics of, 100–01, 101, 102–03
  cognitive-behavioral component of, 102, 124
  definition of, 99
  maladaptive symptom-related behaviors in patients with FAPS, 100
  physical examination for, 99–100
  Rome III diagnostic criteria for adults, 190
  sensory-discrimination component of, 102, 123–24
  See also functional abdominal pain syndrome (FAPS), treatment of
functional abdominal pain syndrome (FAPS), treatment of, 101, 102–03, 156–58
  acupuncture, 157
  medications
    analgesics, 157
    tricyclic antidepressants, 156–57
    tricyclic antidepressants with an SSRI, 157, 169
  psychological therapy, 157

Rome III diagnostic criteria for adults, 190
spinal manipulation, 157
transcutaneous electrical nerve stimulation (TENS), 157
functional anorectal disorders, 88–93
functional anorectal pain, 91
   chronic proctalgia, 91
   levator ani syndrome, 91
   proctalgia fugax, 13, 25, 33, 91–92, 142, 160
   unspecified anorectal pain, 91
functional fecal incontinence, 88–91
   causes of, *89*
   Rome III diagnostic criteria for adults, 191
   nocturnal incontinence, 89
   "organic"/"functional" distinction, 88
   and rectal sensitivity, 90
   and urge incontinence, 90
   See also functional anorectal disorders, treatment of; functional defecation disorders
functional anorectal disorders, treatment of, 159–61
   of functional fecal incontinence, 159–60
      alosetron, 159
      biofeedback, 159
      colostomy, 160
      diphenoxylate with atropine (Lomotil), 159
      loperamide, 159
      sacral nerve stimulation, 160
   of proctalgia fugax, 160
   salbutamol, 160
functional bloating, 98–99
   definition of, 98
   explanations of, 98
      depression of the diaphragm, 98
      excess lumbar lordosis, 98
      hysteria, 98
      protrusion of the abdomen, 98
      and gas distension of the abdomen, 98, 99
   Rome III diagnostic criteria for adults, 188
   See also functional bloating, treatment of
functional bloating, treatment of, 98–99, 153–54
   and diet, 153
   medications, 154
      pancreatic enzymes, 154
      simethicone, 154
      tegaserod, 154
functional bowel disorder (unspecified), *Rome III* diagnostic criteria for adults, 189
functional constipation, 60–67, 92
   acute, 64
   causes of, *63*, 65–67
      dietary considerations, 66
      intestinal motility, 65–66
      psychological, 66–67
   chronic, 64, 71
   definition of, 60, 61
   diagnoses to consider other than functional constipation, 62, *63*, 64
   and systemic diseases, 62, 64
   diagnosis of, 60–62
   drugs as a cause of, 64
   investigation of symptoms, 64–65
   and transit time, 60, 60n, 65
   prevalence of, 60
   Rome III diagnostic criteria for adults, *61, 62,* 189
   See also functional constipation, treatment of
functional constipation, treatment of, *63,* 67, 154–55
   fiber supplementation, 154–55
      methylcellulose (Citrucel), 155
      oat or wheat bran, 154
      polycarbophil (Konsyl; Equalactin), 155
      psyllium (ispaghula [Metamucil]), 154
   laxatives, 155
      bisacodyl, 155
      lubiprostone (Amitiza), 155

functional constipation, treatment of, laxatives *(continued)*
   milk of magnesia, 155
   misoprostil (Cytotec), 155
   polyethylene glycol, 155
   See also enemas
functional defecation disorders, 64
  dyssynergic defecation, 25, 64, 65, 67, 92–93
  inadequate defecatory propulsion, 64, 65, 93
  Rome III diagnostic criteria for adults, 193
  treatment of with biofeedback, 160–61
functional diarrhea, 68–73
  absence of pain in, 68–69
  and alcohol, 69
  and bile salts, 70
  causes of, *69*, 72
  definition of, 68
  diagnoses other than functional diarrhea to consider, 69–71
  diagnosis of, 68–69, *69*
  and diet, 69
  drugs as a cause of, 70
  investigation of symptoms, 71–72
  prevalence of, 68
  Rome III diagnostic criteria for adults, 189
  See also functional diarrhea, treatment of
functional diarrhea, treatment of, 155–56
  alosetron, 156
  cholestyramine, 156
  and diet, 156
  opioids, 156
    codeine, 156
    diphenoxylate (Lomotil), 156
    loperamide, 156
    tincture of opium, 156
functional disorders, 4
  "functional" versus "organic" disorders, 5, 6–7, 9, 11
functional dyspepsia (nonulcer dyspepsia), 74–81, 148, 201
  background of, 74–75
  causes of, 79–81
    chronic gastritis, 80
    drugs, 78
    duodenitis, 80
    gastric acid secretion, 79–80
    gastroduodenal dysmotility, 79
    gastroduodenal hypersensitivity, 80
    Helicobacter pylori, 80
    psychopathological, 80
  and comorbid disease, 79
  definition of, 43, 74, 75
  diagnoses other than functional dyspepsia to consider, 78
  diagnosis of, 75–77
  dyspepsia subgroups, 75
  epidemiology of, 77–78
  prevalence of, 77
  Rome III diagnostic criteria for adults, *77*, 185
  symptoms of, *76*
  treatment of, 147, 148–49
functional esophageal disorders, 82–87
  chest pain of presumed esophageal origin, 83–85
    diagnostic tests for, 84
    and psychiatric comorbidity, 85
    Rome III diagnostic criteria for adults, 184
  functional dysphagia, 85–86, *85*
    investigation of symptoms, 86
    Rome III diagnostic criteria for adults, 184
  functional heartburn, 82–83
    Rome III diagnostic criteria for adults, 184
  globus, 13, 33, 86, 87, 142
    Rome III diagnostic criteria for adults, 185
  motility abnormalities, 85
    diffuse esophageal spasm, 85
    nutcracker esophagus, 85
    testing for, 205

See also functional esophageal disorders, treatment of
functional esophageal disorders, treatment of, 145–47
  of functional chest pain of esophageal origin, 146–47
    antidepressants (sertraline), 146
    anticholinergics (dicyclomine), 146
    behavioral therapy, 146–147
    botulinum toxin, 146
    calcium-channel blockers (nifedipine), 146
    and cognitive behavioral therapy, 147
  of functional dysphagia, 147
    botulinum toxin, 146
  of functional heartburn, 145–36
    acid suppression with histamine$_2$ (H$_2$) receptor antagonist, 145
    acid suppression with proton pump inhibitors (PPIs), 145
    antidepressants, 146
  of globus, 147
functional gallbladder disorders, 25, 103–04
  Rome III diagnostic criteria for adults, 190
  symptoms of, 103
  treatment of, 158
    cholecystectomy, 158
functional gastroduodenal disorders, treatment of, 147–51
  alternative medicine, 150
  antacid/antisecretory medications, 148
    calcium carbonate (TUMS), 148
    proton pump inhibitors (PPIs), 148
  and diet, 148
  eradication of *H. pylori* infection, 148
  hypnotherapy, 149, 153
  miscellaneous medications, 149
    bismuth citrate (DeNol), 149
    dicyclomine (Bentyl, Bentylol), 149
    trimebutine (Modulon), 149
  prokinetic medications, 148–49
    cisapride, 148–49
    domperidone (Motilium), 148
    erythromycin, 149
    metoclopramide, 148
    tegaserod (Zelnorm), 149
  psychotherapy, 149
  See also postprandial distress syndrome (PDS)
functional gastrointestinal disorders (FGIDs), xv–xvi, 4, 8–9, *10*, 24, 28, 62, 82, 99, 127, 177, 181
  classification of, 31, 41
  diagnostic criteria for, 12–13, 184–99
  epidemiologic perspective of, 17, *18*
  and the "hypersensitive" gut, 29
  prevalence of, 13, *14–15*, 16, 19
    according to gender, *16*
    data limitations concerning, 16–17
  and quality of life (QOL), 110–11, 113, 114, 135
  support groups, 225–26
  symptoms of, 143
  See also functional gastrointestinal disorders (FGIDs), causes of; functional gastrointestinal disorders, diagnosis of; functional gastrointestinal disorders, psychological treatments for; functional gastrointestinal disorders, tests for the investigation of; functional gastrointestinal disorders, treatment and management of; *Rome III* diagnostic criteria for children and adolescents with functional gastrointestinal disorders; *Rome III* diagnostic criteria for infants and toddlers with functional gastrointestinal disorders

functional gastrointestinal disorders
(FGIDs), causes of, 32–39
  theoretical causes, 32
    environmental theories, 35–36
    food allergies, 36
    inflammation and bacteriological
      theories, 36–37
    nurture versus nature theories,
      35
    physiological theories, 32–34
    psychosocial theories, 34–35
    visceral hypersensitivity
      theories, 32, 37–38, 59, 83,
      84–85
functional gastrointestinal disorders
(FGIDs), diagnosis of, 43–48
  alarm symptoms
    physical, 46
    psychological, 47
  diagnostic criteria for, 184–99
  follow-up visits after initial diagnosis, 48
  importance of a diagnosis, 44–45
  making a diagnosis, 45
    investigation, 47
    medical history, 45–46
    physical examination, 46–47
  and psychological comorbidity, 48
functional gastrointestinal disorders
(FGIDs), psychological treatments for, 172–74
  cognitive behavioral therapy (CBT),
    172, 173
  dynamic psychotherapy, 173
  hypnotherapy, 173–74
  relaxation training and biofeedback, 172–73
functional gastrointestinal disorders
(FGIDs), tests for the investigation of, 111–12, 114; 200–06
  ambulatory twenty-four-hour pH
    monitoring, 205
  anorectal manometry, 90, 205–06
  endoscopy, 86, 201–03
    aftercare, 203
    colonoscopy/sigmoidoscopy,
      201–02
    endoscopic retrograde
      cholangeopancreatography
      (ERCP), 104, 105, 158, 201
    enteroscopy, 201
    esophagogastroduodenoscopy
      (EGD), 200–01
    precautions, 202–03
    and sedation, 203
  imaging procedures, 203–06
    abdominal ultrasound, 204
    barium studies, 203–04
    computed tomography (CT), 53,
      98, 204
    endoscopic ultrasound, 204
    magnetic resonance imaging
      (MRI), 53, 90, 204
  for esophageal motility, 205
functional gastrointestinal disorders
(FGIDs), treatment and management of, 108–15, 142–43
  appropriate treatment measures,
    113–14
  diagnostic testing, 111–12, 114
  explanation of and reassurance for
    patients, 112–13
  and functional somatic syndromes,
    109, *110*
  and health-related quality of life
    (HRQOL), 110–11, 135
  making a confident diagnosis, 112,
    114
  and medical history, 109–10
  and psychosocial history, 111
  reasons for patient visits, *109*
  See also therapeutic relationship
functional magnetic resonance imaging ($_f$MRI), 58
functional sphincter of Oddi (SO)
  disorders, 103–05
  biliary SO disorder, 104–05
    Rome III diagnostic criteria for
      adults, 191
  pancreatic SO disorder, 105
    Rome III diagnostic criteria for
      adults, 191
  treatment of functional biliary SO
    disorder, 158

botulinum toxin, 158
endoscopic sphincterotomy, 158
nifedipine, 158
nitroglycerine, 158
treatment of pancreatic SO disorder, 158–59

galactose, 22
gallbladder (GB), 24, *25*. *See also* functional gallbladder disorders
gallstones, 204
gastric antrum, 30
gastritis, 22
gastrocolonic response, 35
Gastroenterology International, xvi
gastroesophageal reflux disease (GERD), 75, 81, 82, 94, 97, 145, 147, 163
treatment of, 164, 165, 166
gastroparesis, 97
Giardia lamblia, 55
giardiasis, 70
glucose, 22, 154
Guidelines for the Management of IBS, xv
gut anatomy, function, and physiology, 20
of the anorectum, *25*, 26
effects of emotion on gut function, 29
of the esophagus, 20–21, *21*, 30
lower esophageal sphincter (LES), 20–21, *21*, 28, 166
upper esophageal sphincter, 20
of the gastroduodenum, 21–22, *21*
duodenum, 22, 24
and the production of acid, 22
pylorus, 21–22, 24, 30
stomach, 21
gut motor function, 30–31
of the intestines, 22–24, *23*
cecum, 23
duodenum, 22, 79
ileocecal valve, 23, 24, 30

ileum, 22
jejunum, 22, 24
large intestine/colon, 22, 23
small intestine, 22–23, 30
smooth muscle, 22
water absorption/exchange in, 23–24
of the pancreatic and biliary systems, 24, *25*, 26
gallbladder, 24, *25*
pancreas, 24, *25*
sphincter of Oddi, 24, *25*

health-related quality of life (HRQOL), 110–11, 135
heartburn, 20–21, 77, 163. *See also* functional esophageal disorders
Heaton, Kenneth W., xv, 13
Helicobacter pylori, 8, 22, 56, 78, 80, 164
eradication of, 165
hemoglobin, 24
herbal medicines, 113
Hirschsprung's disease, 33, 65, 206
hydrogen, 24, 54, 98
hyperalgesia, 29, 34, 37
hyperthyroidism, 62

illness, 9, 11. *See also* disease/illness distinction
inflammatory bowel disease (IBD), 54, 69, 70–71, 72
International Congress of Gastroenterology (1984), xv
International Congress of Gastroenterology (1988), xv
International Foundation for Functional Gastrointestinal Disorders (IFFGD), 225
intestines, 22–24, *23*, 35
amount of bacteria in, 24
complex terminology of, 22
gas content of, 98
inflammation of, 36–37
intestinal motility, 57–58
intestinal transit time, 60, 62, 64, 65

236   Index

intestines, *(continued)*
    segments of, 23
    as the site of functional bowel disorders, 24
    large intestine/colon, 37, 53–54, 201–02
    small intestine, 37, 71
    water exchange in and out of, 23
    See also gut anatomy, function, and physiology: of the intestines
Irritable Bowel Symptom Severity Scale, 135
irritable bowel syndrome (IBS), xv, 9, 13, 32, 33, 37, 68, 77, 85, 98, 130, 133, 177, 202
    causes of, 56–59, 166
        intestinal motility, 57–58
        overview of, 56–57
        psychopathology, 58
        visceral hypersensitivity, 59
    in children, 35
    with diarrhea (IBS-D), 68
    lack of medical consensus concerning cause of, xv
    medical costs on in the United States, 49
    and the pain of altered defecation, 62
    prevalence of, *14*, 16, *18*, 49
    and psychological disturbances, 56
    research publications concerning, xvi, *xvi*
    Rome III diagnostic criteria for adults, 188
    severity of, *18*
    See also irritable bowel syndrome (IBS), diagnosis of; irritable bowel syndrome (IBS), treatment of
irritable bowel syndrome (IBS), diagnosis of, 49–59
    alarm symptoms, 50–51, *51*
    alternator IBS (IBS-A), 52
    and comorbid diseases, 56
    diagnoses to consider other than IBS, 53–55
    diagnostic criteria, *50*
    IBS with constipation (IBS-C), 50, 52, *52*, *53*
    IBS with diarrhea (IBS-D), 50, 52, *52*, *53*
    investigation of symptoms, 55
    mixed IBS, 52, *52*, *53*
    and stool form, 51–52, *51*, *53*
    subtypes of, 52–53, *52*, *53*
    symptoms of, 49–51
        abdominal pain, 49–50
        and "pelvic pain," 50
    unsubtyped IBS, 52, *52*, *53*
irritable bowel syndrome (IBS), treatment of, 143, 151–53, 169
    antibiotics, 153
    antidepressants, 152
        alosetron (Lotronex), 152
        desipramine, 152
    approved drugs for, *144*
    and changing of the bacterial flora, 152–53
        and *Bifidobacterium infantis*, 152–53
        and *Clostridium difficile*, 153
        and Rixaximin, 153
    chloride channel activators (lubiprostone), 152
    commercial fiber products containing psyllium (ispaghula), 151
    and the laxative effect of tegaserod (Zelnorm), 152
    loperamide (Imodium), 151
    smooth-muscle relaxants, 151–52
    psychological and behavioral, 153
Irritable Bowel Syndrome (IBS) Network, 225

jejunum, 36, 99
    jejunal gas, 99
    proximal, 204

Klein, K. B., 9
Kruis, Wolfgang, xv

lactase, 36, 54
lactose, 24, 36

digestion of, 22
intolerance of (malabsorption), 54, 72
lactulose, 171
Laetrile, 128
laxatives, 61, 130, 168
　abuse of, 71
　laxative-induced melanosis coli, 72
　See also drugs: laxatives
levator ani muscle, 90, 91, 160
levator ani syndrome, 10, 15, 91, 160
　Rome III diagnostic criteria for adults, 192
liver, 24
liver function tests (LFTs), 103

magnetic resonance imaging (MRI), 53, 90, 204
　See also functional magnetic resonance imaging (fMRI)
mannitol, 171
Marshall, Barry J., 8
methane, 24, 98
methylcellulose, 99
migraine, 95, 96, 156
monosaccharide sugars, 22, 24, 54
motility, 5, 22, 33
　abnormalities of gallbladder and sphincter of Oddi motility, 103–04
　esophageal, 85, 205
　intestinal, 57–58, 65–66
mucosa, 27, 79
mucosal plexus, 27
Munchausen's syndrome, 71

nausea/vomiting disorders, 34, 95, 96–97
　chronic idiopathic nausea, 95
　　Rome III diagnostic criteria for adults, 187
　　treatment of, 150
　cyclic vomiting syndrome (CVS), 95
　　Rome III diagnostic criteria for adults, 187
　　treatment of, 151
　functional vomiting, 95
　　Rome III diagnostic criteria for adults, 187
　　treatment of, 150
　prevalence of, 95
neurogastroenterology, 25–26
neuropeptides, 5
neurotransmitters, 28, 28, 33, 179
　dopamine, 166
　See also serotonin
nitrogen, 98
Norton, Nancy, xvii

"organic" vs. "functional" disorders, 5, 6–7, 9, 11
oxygen, 98

pancreas, 24, 25, 70
　cancer of, 78
　pancreatic enzymes, 103, 105
pancreatitis, 103, 105, 158
Parkinson's disease, 64
peptic ulcers, 4, 5–6, 6, 36, 163
　asymptomatic, 6
　diagnosis of, 5, 43
　and excessive stomach acid, 7–8, 22
　and "nonulcer" dyspepsia, 5, 6
peristalsis, 20, 30, 30, 96
　esophageal, 205
placebo effect, 116, 117, 118, 120, 120–21, 125, 128, 131–32
　Cochrane meta-analysis of placebo-controlled trials, 148
　and the doctor as the placebo, 123
　optimization of, 123
　placebo response, 112, 132
positron emission tomography (PET), 58
postherpetic neuralgia, 156
postprandial distress syndrome (PDS), 75, 81, 147
　response of to medication, 149
　Rome III diagnostic criteria for adults, 185
premenstrual syndrome (PMS), 98

probiotics. *See* drugs: probiotics
"problem patients," 9
proctalgia fugax, 13, 25, 33, 142, 160
   Rome III diagnostic criteria for adults, 192
prostaglandin-inhibiting aspirin, 78
proton pump inhibitors (PPIs), 83, 84, 85, 145, 148, 151, 163, 164
psychopathology, 58, 99
psyllium, 99, 151, 154
puborectalis muscle, 25, 90

quality of life (QOL), 110–11, 113, 114, 135
   disease-specific, 135
   health-related, 110–11, 135

randomized clinical trials (RCTs), 116, 118, 120–21, 124–25, 127, 141, 156
   analysis and reporting of, 135, *136–37, 138*, 138
   and the CONSORT guidelines, 135, *136–37*, 138
   meta-analysis and systematic reviews, 140
   and bias, 128–29, *129*
   elements of, 129–39
      blinding (double-blinding), randomization, and control treatments, 131–32
      hypotheses and outcomes, 130
   ethical issues concerning, 138–39
   and evidence-based medicine, 139–40
      advantages of, 139
      limitations of, 140
   need for, 127–28
   outcome assessment, 133, 135
      binary scale, 133, 134
      measuring RCT outcome, *134*
      visual analogue scale (VAS), 133, *134*, 135
   patient selection and characteristics, 130–31
   and the placebo effect, 131–32
   trial and conduct of, 132–33
      crossover design, 132
      intention-to-treat analysis, 133
      parallel group study design, 132
      superiority or noninferiority trial, 132–33
rectum, 23, 25, *26,* 33, 90
reductionism, 7
research, 178–79
   and the importance of communication between disciplines, 179–81
   See also randomized clinical trials (RCTs)
Rome Foundation, xvi–xvii
Rome I: The Functional Gastrointestinal Disorders (1994), xvi, 13
Rome II: The Functional Gastrointestinal Disorders (2000), xvi, 13, 95
Rome III: The Functional Gastrointestinal Disorders (2006), xvii, xvii, 4, 9, 13, 16, 26, 50, 67, 129, 145, 177
   definition of functional abdominal pain syndrome, 99
   definition of functional anorectal disorders, 88
   definition of functional bloating, 98
   definition of functional constipation, 60, 61
   definition of functional diarrhea, 68
   definition of functional dyspepsia, 74
   definitions of functional esophageal disorders, 82, 83, 85
   definition of globus, 86, 87
   definition of irritable bowel syndrome, 49
   diagnosis criteria of, 44
   guidelines for a therapeutic relationship, 121, *122*
   rejection of psychosomatic theory in, 58
   suggestions of for the study of cellular and neural mechanisms, 179

See also *Rome III* diagnostic criteria for children and adolescents with functional gastrointestinal disorders; *Rome III* diagnostic criteria for infants and toddlers with functional gastrointestinal disorders
Rome III diagnostic criteria for adults with functional gastrointestinal disorders, 184–193
Rome III diagnostic criteria for children and adolescents with functional gastrointestinal disorders, 196–97
rumination syndrome, 96–98
    prevalence of in young women, 97
    Rome III diagnostic criteria for adults, 188
    treatment of with proton pump inhibitors (PPIs), 151

scleroderma, 89
secretomotor nerves, 27
sensory nerve fibers, 27–28
serotonin, 26, 31, 33–34, 179
    serotonin (5-HT), 155
    serotonin analogues, 155, 168
SF-36 (Short Form of the General Health Questionnaire), 135
Shigella, 37
Sickness Impact Profile, 135
sphincter of Oddi, 24, *25*
    disorders of, 25
    and external anal sphincter weakness, 90
    See also functional sphincter of Oddi disorders
sorbitol, 171
statistical analysis, 135, 138
    and the Bonferroni correction, 138
    and the intention-to-treat (ITT) principle, 138
steatorrhea, 70
stomach, 30, 35, 79, 201, 204
    cancer of, 78
stool/feces, 23, 24
    fecal impaction, 90
    retention of (encopresis), 66, 90
    See also Bristol Stool Form Scale; constipation; diarrhea; functional anorectal disorders; functional constipation; functional diarrhea
symptoms, 3
    chronic, 3–4
    functional, 6–7
    and pathology, 4–5
    personal nature of, 3
    without pathology, 5
syndrome, 3, 9

therapeutic relationship, 108–09, 116–25
    components of, 116, *117*, 118
    and evidence-based medicine, 124–25
    guidelines for, 121, *122*, 124
    importance of a diagnosis to the patient, *119*, 123
    and the natural history of the disease, 118
    and the nocebo effect, 121
    and pain relief, 123–24
    and the placebo effect, 116, *117*, 118, *120*, 120–21, 125
    and the doctor as the placebo, 123
    optimization of, 123
    and the power of a positive message, 118, *119*
    promotion of, 179
    and the therapeutic equation, 118, 120–21
    and therapeutic gain, 116, *117*, 138
    workings of, 122–24
Torsoli, Aldo, xv
transcendental meditation, 172–73
transit time. See intestines: intestinal transit time

ulcerative colitis, 54, 201

Understanding the Irritable Gut, xvi, 4, 183
University of North Carolina Center for Functional GI and Motility Disorders, 225
U.S. Food and Drug Administration, 128, 143, 167, 171

venesection, 128
vomiting. *See* nausea/vomiting disorders

villous adenoma, 71, 72
visceral hyperalgesia, 34
visceral hypersensitivity, 32, 59, 83, 84–85
 theories of, 37–38

Warren, J. Robin, 8
waste pigments, 24
Whitehead, William, xvii

yoga, 172–73